Ethical Challenges for Military Health Care Personnel

Dealing with Epidemics

W0113501

**Edited by Daniel Messelken
and David Winkler**

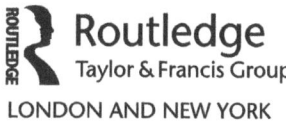

Routledge
Taylor & Francis Group

LONDON AND NEW YORK

First published 2018
by Routledge

2 Park Square, Milton Park, Abingdon, Oxfordshire OX14 4RN
52 Vanderbilt Avenue, New York, NY 10017

Routledge is an imprint of the Taylor & Francis Group, an informa business

First issued in paperback 2020

British Library Cataloguing in Publication Data
A catalogue record for this book is available from the British Library

Library of Congress Cataloging in Publication Data
A catalog record for this book has been requested

ISBN: 978-1-4724-8073-6 (hbk)
ISBN: 978-0-367-59425-1 (pbk)

Typeset in Times New Roman
by Wearset Ltd, Boldon, Tyne and Wear

Contents

Contributors

Cécile M. Bensimon is Director of Ethics and Professional Affairs at the Canadian Medical Association and an adjunct professor in the Faculty of Health Sciences at the University of Ottawa. Cécile earned her PhD from the Institute of Medical Science at the University of Toronto. Previously, she was at the University of Toronto Leslie Dan Faculty of Pharmacy and Faculty of Dentistry after returning from a visiting scholarship at Tel Aviv University's Sackler School of Medicine in humanitarian and disaster ethics. Dr Bensimon completed a post-doctoral fellowship at the University of Toronto Joint Centre for Bioethics. Her publications have appeared in the *British Journal of Psychiatry*, the *Journal of the American College of Surgeons*, the *Journal of Bioethical Inquiry*, *Public Health Ethics* and *Social Science and Medicine*.

Lizzy Bernthal is a registered general nurse and midwife and senior research fellow within the Medical Directorate, Birmingham, UK. She is a qualitative researcher and is passionate about supporting clinicians' psychological resilience, empowerment and ethical decision-making. She teaches evidence-based practice and ethics and is an active member of the International Committee of Military Medicine workshop regarding ethical decision-making. She is editorial member of three health journals, including membership of the international advisory board and guest editor of the first nursing edition of the *Journal of the Royal Army Medical Corps* (published in December 2015). She was appointed an honorary research fellow at the University of Southampton in 2012 and at King's College London in 2014, and a senior lecturer at the University of Birmingham in 2016.

Philippe Calain is Director of Research at the Research Unit on Humanitarian Stakes and Practices (UREPH), MSF Switzerland. As a medical doctor, he specialized in infectious diseases, virology and tropical medicine. After several years of clinical activities in Belgium and Switzerland, he joined the Department of Microbiology at the University of Geneva, where he received a doctorate in biology in 1995. He was appointed as a virologist at the US-CDC from 1995 until 1997. He later worked in Rwanda (ICRC), Afghanistan (MSF) and Laos (WHO). He served as an external member of the WHO Research Ethics Review Committee in 2010–13. He has published peer-reviewed papers on humanitarian ethics, public health ethics, global health governance, public health surveillance and extractive industries.

Heather Draper was appointed to a newly created chair in bioethics at the University of Warwick in January 2017. She is widely published and a recognised expert in several research fields. Relevant to this collection, she was lead investigator on the 'Military Healthcare professionals' experience of ethical challenges while on Ebola humanitarian deployment (Sierra Leone)' project and again on a project evaluating an ethical decision-making tool (the four-quadrant approach) in a Role Three hospital. She was co-investigator on a project exploring the ethical issues faced by deployed medical directors. She was Vice Chair of the COST action Disaster Bioethics (2012–16). Professor Draper is a member of the UK Defence Medical Service Ethics Committee and ethics consultant to the Royal Centre for Defence Medicine's programme of research on military medical ethics.

Paul Eagan is a public health physician in the Royal Canadian Medical Service. He is the current head of the communicable disease control section and acting director of the Directorate of Force Health Protection, Canadian Forces Health Services Group. He holds a medical degree from the University of Calgary and has done postgraduate medical training in family medicine, obstetrics, gynaecology and preventive medicine. He holds specialist certification with the Canadian College of Family Physicians, the American Board of Preventive Medicine and the Royal College of Physicians and Surgeons of Canada. He has extensive clinical experience in resource-scarce medical situations in Canada's north. He has worked in Afghanistan building health system capacity and was instrumental in establishing the postgraduate residency programme in infectious disease and preventive medicine for the Government of Afghanistan. He has played a significant role in formulating and delivering the Canadian Armed Forces response to the Ebola epidemic and has contributed to NATO doctrine on the subject.

Sheena M. Eagan received her PhD in the medical humanities from the Institute for the Medical Humanities at the University of Texas Medical Branch and her Master of Public Health (MPH) at the Uniformed Services University of the Health Sciences. Dr Eagan's areas of research and teaching include military medical ethics, the philosophy of medicine, public health ethics, the history of medicine and the medical humanities. She has presented academic papers at conferences in the humanities, medical ethics and military history in North America, Europe and Asia. Currently, Dr Eagan is an assistant professor in the Department of Bioethics and Interdisciplinary Studies at East Carolina University.

Chris Gibson (MBE) joined the Army in 1984 and served until 2004 with the Royal Military Police. His service during that period was predominantly with the Close Protection Unit, where he undertook numerous operational deployments. He commissioned into the Royal Army Medical Corps in 2004 and has seen service with a close support medical regiment as a welfare, training and operations officer. Further postings have included as an exchange officer in Canada, where he focused principally on improving Canadian Professionally Qualified Officer training. A graduate of the NHS Staff College, he enjoyed developing and delivering a portfolio of leadership development courses for NHS executives. His assignment to the Army Medical Services Training Centre afforded him the opportunity to utilise his postgraduate qualifications in simulation, management and leadership to assist in best preparing units for operational deployment. This included the demands of developing a methodology for training and assuring all those who deployed to West Africa to assist in tackling the Ebola virus disease outbreak. Of late he was tasked by the government to assist the London Ambulance Service NHS Trust to come out of CQC-imposed special measures. Widowed, he has two boys, Ethan (16) and Lewis (15), who attend a local boarding school.

Paul Gilbert is Emeritus Professor of Philosophy at the University of Hull, UK. His current research interests are principally in military ethics and the ethics of roles more generally. His most recent books are *An Introduction to Metaphilosophy* (with S. Overgaard and S. Burwood, Cambridge University Press, 2013) and *Cultural Identity and Political Ethics* (Edinburgh University Press, 2010).

Catherine Hale is an influential legal expert on issues related to health care, particularly current or topical ethical issues. As a regular speaker at external events and media commentator she has provided lectures and commentary on key health care and legal issues. Catherine's research interests include ethical values within medicine and professionalism, as well as ethics in and conflict and disaster medicine.

Jeremy Henning is currently the Defence Consultant Advisor in Critical Care Medicine to the UK Armed Forces. He is a serving officer and an intensive care consultant, who carries out his day-to-day clinical work in north-east England. He is the veteran of many military operations, from warfighting to counter-insurgency, from humanitarian action to disaster relief. He has been the medical director of a field hospital on one tour of duty. His most recent tour was in Sierra Leone. He has wide ranging interests within critical care medicine, from researching basic science of hypovolaemia to lecturing on human factors and leadership. His multiple operational tours have exposed him to multiple ethical issues, which have made him a keen student in this field as well.

Jillian Horning is a graduate of the MSc in Global Health programme and the Honours Bachelor of Arts and Science programme at McMaster University. She specialized in moral distress, bioethics and psychology, with a concentration on mental health in the population of military health care providers. Her research interests include moral injury and distress, psychological stress processes and atypically stressful work environments, as well as psychological resilience, mindfulness and spiritual health.

Matthew Hunt is the Director of Research and an associate professor in the McGill University School of Physical and Occupational Therapy, and an associate member of the McGill Biomedical Ethics Unit and Institute for Health and Social Policy. Matthew's research interests are at the intersections of ethics, global health and rehabilitation. He currently leads research projects related to palliative care in humanitarian emergencies, oversight of research in situations of disaster and ethics of humanitarian health care and public health responses. Matthew also heads a capacity building project for rehabilitation providers in Haiti and co-leads the Humanitarian Health Ethics Research Group (http://humanitarianhealthethics.net).

Christian Janke is a specialist in tropical medicine and epidemiology. He was the senior medical officer and commander of the German armed forces detachment in Liberia during the 2014–15 Ebola outbreak. Since he left the Bundeswehr in 2016, he has been a freelancing consultant for global public health and still works in Liberia, among other places. Recently, he has been the medical project manager for the European Medical Corps Isolation Hospital Project operated by the German Red Cross.

Simon Jenkins is Senior Teaching Fellow at the University of Warwick. He specialises in medical ethics, having completed his PhD on the ethics of sperm and egg allocation at the University of Birmingham. He is a philosopher and bioethicist with expertise in qualitative methods and methodologies. His academic interests include: Ebola virus disease, military medicine, social robotics in health, environmental ethics, reproductive ethics, informed consent, research ethics and epistemology. He is co-chair of Effective Altruism: Birmingham, a local chapter of an organization that applies maximizing consequentialist principles to everyday life.

Ivan Kholikov is a graduate of the Military University, Moscow. He participated in such international campaigns as the United Nations Mission in Angola (UNAVEM III), 1996, the Multinational Operation in Kosovo (KFOR), 2001, and the United Nations Mission in Chad (MINURCAT), 2009. Currently he holds the position of Chief of the International Cooperation Branch of the Main Military Medical Directorate of the Russian Federation Defence Ministry. In 2014, he was a leader of the Russian military Ebola response team in the Republic of Guinea. Dr Kholikov holds a PhD and is a professor in international law and the author of numerous publications on peacekeeping, international humanitarian law and cooperation in the field of military medicine. He has also been a member of international teaching staff of the ICMM Law of Armed Conflict (LOAC) courses since 2010 and is the legal advisor to the secretary general of the ICMM. Dr Kholikov has been decorated with a number of awards and medals for distinguished service.

Ana Komparic is a PhD candidate in pharmaceutical sciences and collaborative specialization in bioethics at the University of Toronto, Canada. Her background is in bioethics, the philosophy of science and immunology. Her primary research interests concern the philosophy and policy of health and pharmaceutical insurance and pharmacovigilance, as well as public health ethics, global health ethics and applied ethics more broadly.

Daniel Messelken is a research associate at the Center for Ethics at Zurich University and leader of the Zurich Center for Military Medical Ethics (www. cmme.uzh.ch). He also serves as Head Ethics Teacher for the Center of Reference for Education on IHL and Ethics of the International Committee of Military Medicine and is member of the Board of Directors of the International Society for Military Ethics in Europe (EuroISME). Dr Messelken studied philosophy and political science in Leipzig and Paris (1998–2004) and received his PhD in philosophy from the University of Leipzig in 2010. Besides military medical ethics, his main research fields include just war theory, the morality of violence, military ethics and applied ethics more generally.

Marc Poncin is a researcher and humanitarian expert at the Research Unit on Humanitarian Stakes and Practices (UREPH), Médecins Sans Frontières, Switzerland. He began his career as a researcher in structural biology after obtaining a PhD in molecular biophysics from Paris 7 University. He joined MSF in 1995 and has in the intervening years worked extensively in Africa as emergency coordinator and head of various missions. He also served as Deputy Director General and Head of Programs of the Swiss branch of MSF. During the Ebola crisis, he served as the coordinator of the MSF response in Guinea from April to December 2014.

Kira Sazonova is a PhD candidate in international law and a PhD candidate in international relations. Currently she holds a position of Associate Professor at the Russian Presidential Academy of National Economy and Public Administration. She won the Grant of the President of the Russian Federation for young scientists in 2010 and the Grant of the Institute for Public Planning for the socially important research in 2011. Being a member of the Russian Association of International Law and the author of more than 120 scientific publications on international law and international relations, she is also a permanent expert of Russian media in international law.

Lisa Schwartz is the Arnold L. Johnson Chair in Health Care Ethics in the Faculty of Health Sciences at McMaster University, Full Professor in the Department of Clinical Epidemiology and Biostatistics, Director of the PhD in Health Policy, Co-associate Director of the Centre for Health Economics and Policy Analysis (CHEPA) and an associate member of the Department of Philosophy. She is also the Vice Chair of the Standing Committee on Ethics at the Canadian Institutes of Health Research (CIHR) and a member of the Ethics Committee at the Royal College of Physicians and Surgeons of Canada. In 2014, she joined the Médecins Sans Frontières (MSF) Ethics Review Board. Dr Schwartz's research background is in ethics and human research, evaluation of ethics education in medicine and advocacy in health care. She is the primary investigator on CIHR-funded studies examining the ethical challenges faced by health care professionals (civilian and military) providing humanitarian health care assistance abroad and on ethics and policy development in humanitarian health care agencies. Dr Schwartz has collaborated with the International Committee of the Red Cross project on 'Health Care in Danger' and is a member of the World Health Organization's Ethics and Ebola working group.

Bryn Williams-Jones is Full Professor and Director of the bioethics programme (http://espum.umontreal.ca/etudes/domaines-detudes/bioethique/) at the Department of Social and Preventive Medicine, School of Public Health (ESPUM), University of Montreal. An interdisciplinary scholar trained in Bioethics, Dr Williams-Jones is interested in the socio-ethical and policy implications of health innovations in diverse contexts. His work examines the conflicts that arise in academic research and professional practice with a view to developing ethical tools to manage these conflicts when they cannot be avoided. Current projects focus on issues in professional ethics, public health ethics, research integrity and ethics education. Dr Williams-Jones heads the Research Ethics and Integrity Group and is Editor-in-Chief of the open access journal *BioéthiqueOnline* (http://bioethiqueonline.ca).

David T. Winkler is Chairman of the Center of Reference for Education on International Humanitarian Law and Ethics of the International Committee of Military Medicine (www.cimm-icmm.org). He is a medical doctor specializing in neurology and holds a PhD in neurobiology. Lieutenant Colonel Winkler is a staff officer in the Swiss Armed Forces Medical Services Directorate. He conducts clinical and academic work at the University Hospital Basel, Switzerland.

Acknowledgements

This book could not have been completed without the support and help of a number of people, to whom we would like to express our gratitude.

We would first like to profoundly thank our authors, who wrote and revised their chapters thoroughly and with diligence and who were open enough to share their own experiences and knowledge.

We are thankful to Major General (MG) Dr Andreas Stettbacher, MG Dr Roger van Hoof and Prof Peter Schaber, under the patronage of whom the conference was organized during which most of the chapters of this volume were first discussed. Prof Martin Oberholzer is also to be acknowledged for his lasting altruistic support in building the cornerstones of the institutional framework that we work in.

Gratitude is also due to Shazia Islamshah and Jack Richard Williams, who, at different points of time, supported the putting together of the manuscript by conducting initial research on the topic and in proofreading the drafts and revisions of the various chapters.

Finally, we would like to thank the anonymous referee for the constructive comments and helpful suggestions made on earlier versions of the manuscript, as well as Andrew Humphrys and Hannah Ferguson at Routledge for their advice and support throughout the conception and production of this volume.

Introduction to the volume

Daniel Messelken and David T. Winkler

The subject of this book, ethical challenges for (military) health care practitioners during epidemics, is unfortunately of lasting relevance, not only in view of the 2014/15 outbreak of the Ebola virus disease in West Africa but also with regard to the high likelihood of similar and recurring events in the future. Throughout human history, diseases like the plague, cholera, smallpox, or aggressive flu variants have reached epidemic or pandemic levels and killed millions. The increased volume and ease of international travel have increased the speed with which diseases can spread and within recent years SARS, MERS, Zika, and Ebola have all threatened populations (Sands et al., 2016). Despite the fact that epidemic outbreaks of communicable diseases necessitate complex responses that regularly involve military actors with their logistic and medical capabilities, the literature on the topic almost exclusively focuses on civilian efforts in cases of such disasters. However, military actors are often decisively involved if not at the forefront of responding to disasters and large-scale public health emergencies.

This book aims to fill a gap in the literature and amend the discussion of ethical issues in epidemic response and preparedness by adding analyses of the specific aspects that come with the deployment of military assets in the context of epidemic disease outbreaks. It does so by bringing together authors from both academia, with their analytical skills, and contributors who can directly report their experiences in the field as members of military or humanitarian emergency response teams. The dialogue between these quite different authors and their texts has proven productive during the annual workshops of the International Committee of Military Medicine (ICMM) on Military Medical Ethics held in Switzerland and it remains thought-provoking in written form as well.

In our introduction to the volume, we want to first clarify some important (medical) terms and concepts which some readers may not be familiar with. We will then give a short overview on the development of the Ebola disease outbreak in West Africa in 2014/15 before briefly discussing the central ethical issues that arise during epidemics. Finally, we will present the contributions to this volume and show how they interrelate in looking at the topic from different perspectives and with different backgrounds.

Disease, epidemics, and pandemics – some clarifications

Prior to embarking on the discussion, we should start by clarifying some terms that are often used but nevertheless may not be familiar to everyone. This is not only useful to avoid confusion and misunderstanding but will also already help to introduce the context in which the contributions should be read. Of these it is most important to clearly distinguish between infectious diseases, epidemics, and pandemics.

Infectious diseases, according to the WHO, "are caused by pathogenic microorganisms, such as bacteria, viruses, parasites or fungi" and, by definition, "can be spread, directly or indirectly, from one person to another."[1] Nothing is thus implied regarding the severity or the deadliness of the disease and the number of cases that occur. Typical examples of regularly occurring infectious diseases are influenza or salmonellosis. In tropical countries, malaria and dengue fever can be added to the list. Among the most famous and most feared of infectious diseases are plague, smallpox, typhoid, cholera, tuberculosis, and also Ebola.

The occurrence of some cases of an infectious disease alone is not sufficient to talk of an epidemic, neither does an epidemic presuppose an infectious disease. Epidemics are defined, in the *Oxford Dictionary of Epidemiology*, as the "occurrence in a community or region of cases of an illness, specific health-related behaviour, or other health-related events *clearly in excess of normal expectancy*" (Porta, 2014, p. 93, emphasis added). Epidemics are thus essentially defined by the number of cases and not by the nature of the illness.

> The number of cases indicating the presence of an epidemic varies according to the agent, size, and type of population exposed; previous experience or lack of exposure to the disease; and time and place of occurrence. Epidemicity is thus *relative to usual frequency* of the disease in the same area, among the specified population, at the same season of the year.
>
> (Porta, 2014, p. 93, emphasis added)

A similar definition is proposed by the WHO.[2] The important and distinguishing criteria for the occurrence of an epidemic is thus a higher number of cases compared to the usual and expected occurrence of an illness.

In contrast to an epidemic, a pandemic is defined by the larger geographical area that it affects. A pandemic is thus defined as an "epidemic occurring over a very wide area, crossing international boundaries, and usually affecting a large number of people" (Porta, 2014, p. 209). This has indirect consequences on the kind of illnesses that have pandemic potential, as they must be able to spread quickly in order to reach a certain level of geographical coverage. "Characteristics of an infectious agent influencing the causation of a pandemic include: the agent must be able to infect humans, to cause disease in humans, and to spread easily from human to human" (Porta, 2014, p. 209).

Most often, the immediate reaction to epidemics are public health measures that are both planned and executed by the (national) public health systems. Thus, it is usually civilian actors that are on the "front line" and the existing health care system that is relied upon. If the military and their health care services are involved, it is also most of the time on a national level, such as during the SARS or H1N1 crises, where no transnational deployment of military health care personnel were required. This was different during the Ebola outbreak in 2014/15, which resulted in new challenges to the military health services that were involved in the international effort to avert the escalation of the Ebola epidemic to a global pandemic.

The development of the Ebola epidemic in West Africa in 2014–16

The Ebola virus is fortunately only endemic among some species of animals such as certain bats and apes; however, this means that every occurrence of Ebola among human populations has the potential to reach the level of an epidemic as it can be considered to be "in excess of normal expectancy." This is compounded by the fact that the Ebola disease is one of the world's most infectious diseases and spreads easily and quickly after a first infection occurs. The fact that Ebola, like other forms of haemorrhagic fevers, has a very high mortality rate is only relevant with regard to the question of an epidemic insofar as dead bodies remain carriers of the disease and burials of the first victims act as the starting point for Ebola disease epidemics – as was the case in 2014 (Baize et al., 2014). Densely populated areas or communities that live very closely together with poor hygienic standards are also factors that contribute to the spreading of communicable diseases, all of which were present in the affected countries in West Africa. Nevertheless, the massive Ebola disease outbreak in 2014–16 was largely underestimated at the beginning, even by international bodies such as the World Health Organization (WHO).

According to research findings, the 2014–16 Ebola disease epidemic in West Africa started in a small village in the Guéckédou Province of the Republic of Guinea, where a one-year-old infant who had died in December 2013 has been identified as the first victim of the outbreak (Baize et al., 2014). Soon after his death, several family members also showed similar symptoms and some of them passed away. Others who had been close or attended one of the funerals were infected too, and furthered the spread of the disease in the region. It took a while, however, until Ebola was suspected to be the reason for the "mysterious disease characterized by fever, severe diarrhoea, vomiting, and an apparent high fatality rate" (Baize et al., 2014, pp. 1418–1419). Until then, the Ebola disease had never occurred in the West African subcontinent. In early March 2016, regional hospitals alerted the Ministry of Health in Guinea and also Médecins Sans Frontières, which was running a malaria project in the vicinity, and subsequent laboratory investigation proved that the "mysterious disease" was Ebola. As a result, on 21 March 2014 the Guinean Ministry of Health declared an outbreak of the Ebola disease and four days later the WHO stated that it was notified of a rapidly evolving outbreak of Ebola virus disease in forested areas south eastern Guinea.... As of 25 March 2014, a total of 86 suspected cases including 60 deaths (case fatality ratio: 69.7%) had been reported. Four health care workers are among the victims.[3]

Interestingly, the WHO statement ended by saying that the "WHO does not recommend that any travel or trade restrictions be applied to Guinea in respect to this event." By late May 2014, the outbreak had reached Conakry, Guinea's capital, and the disease also spread to neighbouring Liberia and Sierra Leone. On August 8, 2014, the WHO declared that the outbreak had reached the level of a public health emergency of international concern.[4] Case numbers continued to grow, reached their peaked in late 2014, and started to decline thereafter. Contrary to widespread fears, only isolated cases occurred outside the affected region. By June 2016, all affected countries had been declared free of Ebola and, by the time of writing, no new cases have been reported.

Looking back, the Ebola epidemic in 2014–16 was the largest outbreak of the Ebola disease in history. Between 2014 and 2016, more than 28,000 confirmed cases of Ebola occurred and more than 11,000 patients died of Ebola, mainly in Liberia, Guinea, and Sierra Leone, with few cases in neighbouring countries or among expats. In comparison, *all* previous outbreaks of the Ebola disease combined had "only" resulted in 2,427 reported cases and 1,597 fatalities.[5] In addition to these direct victims of the epidemic, there was also an important indirect impact on the health care system and public health in general, which has been neglected in the media coverage. According to the figures of the Centers for Disease Control and Prevention (CDC), more than 500 health care workers in West Africa died of Ebola, which amounts, for example, to an 8 percent loss of the health care workforce in Liberia. As another indirect and rather "hidden" side effect of the concentration of the fight against Ebola, it is estimated that approximately 10,000 additional people died of malaria, tuberculosis, or HIV as a result of the reduced availability of general health care owing to focus on the fight against Ebola. The situation in the affected countries in West Africa did therefore fulfil the criteria of a disaster, which is defined as "a sudden, calamitous event that seriously disrupts the functioning of a community or society and causes human, material, and economic or environmental losses that exceed the community's or society's ability to cope using its own resources."[6]

The epidemic had hit countries with already weak or deficient health care systems that lacked the resilience to cope with the crisis created by the Ebola epidemic. As a result, they were further negatively affected, being unable to cope and requiring external assistance. These severe impacts occurred even though the (international) responses were eventually much bigger and much more organized than during previous occurrences of Ebola. By the end of 2015, more than 3.6 billion US dollars had been spent for Ebola response activities and several countries from around the world had also mobilized and deployed logistical and medical support to the affected region.

One reason why international reaction to the epidemic was eventually so extensive is probably to be found in the strong media attention that the outbreak received. Both the nature of the disease and the potential of a global pandemic were factors that favoured a broad public interest and it is difficult to judge at what point the coverage become a media hype and what would amount to justified coverage. The fear or even panic of a pandemic that spread around the world also led to extensive security measures, for example at airports. The dense and extensive infrastructure of today's interconnected world with frequent and direct flight connections suddenly begun to be seen as a risk factor as not only people but also the virus could travel long distances. In addition, the 2014–16 epidemic did not only occur in a remote jungle but quickly reached cities with international airports. Compared to previous outbreaks of the Ebola disease, the changed international environment, which is now much more interconnected both physically (flight connection) and virtually (social networks), played its role in generating risks and perception. Fortunately, the pessimistic forecasts, which predicted up to 1.4 million Ebola victims (Meltzer et al., 2014, p. 3), did not become a reality.

A remarkable particularity of the 2014–16 epidemic was the large involvement of international military health care providers sent by countries such as Russia, the USA, the UK, and Germany in order to curb the spread of the disease and prevent a pandemic. Interestingly, it may have been the call of an NGO that led to these deployments. In September 2014, Médecins Sans Frontières (MSF), which was the first and, over the whole epidemic, the strongest nonstate actor to respond on the ground,[7] urged the international community to strengthen their support. In a speech to the UN, MSF president Joanne Liu urged "that states immediately deploy *civilian and military assets* with expertise in biohazard containment" (Médecins Sans Frontières, 2015, p. 13, emphasis added). This public appeal for (logistic and medical) support from the *military* is probably unprecedented in the history of MSF and emphasizes how difficult the situation on the ground had become. As a result, a number of (non-African) countries deployed military personnel to take part in specific Ebola missions. It is the involvement of military personnel in the 2014–16 outbreak that differentiates it from other outbreaks and that was the reason for this volume that looks at the challenges that these military actors had to face. For them, these deployments were somehow a new kind of mission as they do not belong to the traditional tasks of the military, even though one might see them as an expanded kind of humanitarian intervention or civil–military cooperation.

Medical aspects of the 2014–16 Ebola epidemic

Epidemics are particularly frightening when provoked by infectious agents that are highly contagious and/or cause a very high fatality rate. Severe epidemics and pandemics have been occurring repeatedly over the last centuries, with outbreaks of smallpox and measles, followed by Russian influenza, Spanish influenza, and the respiratory syndromes MERS (Zumla et al., 2015) and SARS

(Heymann et al., 2015) in more recent years. In most cases, epidemics are caused by a virus spreading from a zoonosis in wild animals to human beings (McCloskey et al., 2014). Filoviruses like the Ebola virus and the Marburg virus have repeatedly caused smaller epidemics in the final quarter of the twentieth century (Bausch et al., 2006). The rapid spreading of the 2014–16 Ebola virus disease outbreak in western Africa caused over 28,616 confirmed cases, 11,310 deaths, and a pandemic threat (WHO, 2016). In this section, we aim at providing basic medical information about the Ebola disease, its pathomechanisms, and current treatment options. This brief overview on the Ebola disease shall seek to clarify the specific threats that this viral disease has to the population in affected areas as well as to health care workers fighting against the spreading of the disease. We may also then better understand the measures that must be taken into account when providing military medical support in Ebola disease epidemics.

The Ebola virus was first isolated after occurrences of haemorrhagic fever syndromes in Zaire (now the Democratic Republic of the Congo) and Sudan (now Republic of South Sudan) in 1976 (WHO/International Study Team, 1978; International Commission, 1978). It is a single-stranded negative-sense RNA virus with five subtypes currently known. While the reservoir of the Makona variant of the Ebola virus responsible for the 2013 outbreak had until then remained unknown, the Ebola virus persists in fruit bats, as well as in the body fluids of an infected person. Human body fluids are the main route of infection responsible for the spreading of the Ebola disease. The Ebola virus is present inter alia in the blood and the urine, and patients may disseminate the viruses by vomiting and diarrhoea (Vetter et al., 2016). Purely airborne viral transmissions (for example by coughing) cannot be excluded, but droplet transmission seems to be very rare. Sexual transmission is rare, but may cause flare-ups after the epidemic, as the Ebola virus can persist for long time periods in the semen of Ebola disease survivors (Mate et al., 2015). The unexpectedly rapid spreading of the virus in 2014 may have been facilitated by a change of the viral structure, increasing its preference for human cells over bat cells (Urbanowicz et al., 2016).

The Ebola virus enters the body via mucosa, skin lesions, or injuries. The Ebola virus first settles in local immune cells at the entry site before spreading into various organs including the liver, the spleen, and lymph nodes (Beeching et al., 2014). The Ebola disease has an incubation time of one to 21 days. Widespread viral expression triggers inflammatory responses, interferon and TNF-alpha production, subsequent loss of the vascular integrity as well as disseminated intravascular coagulation, kidney injury, and hepatic failure.

Clinical symptoms start with fever and malaise, followed by gastrointestinal signs and nonspecific manifestations (such as headache, muscle pain, asthenia, and delirium) lasting from days three to 10 (Chertow et al., 2014). An estimated 30 to 70 percent of patients in the epidemic area showed a fatal outcome, with diminishing consciousness, shock, coma, and death occurring at a median of nine days from onset of symptoms (Beeching et al., 2014; Team, 2014). Recovering patients gradually resolved the gastrointestinal symptoms and regained energy. Patients surviving the initial 13 days of the Ebola disease had a very high rate of survival (Chertow et al., 2014). In a subset of the 17,000 Ebola disease survivors, there is recent evidence of a post-Ebola syndrome with inter alia painful joints and hearing complaints (Burki, 2016; Fowler et al., 2016). The Ebola virus may persist in immune-privileged body sites of Ebola disease survivors, e.g., the eye and the central nervous system, where it also can cause chronic uveitis (Varkey et al., 2015) and meningoencephalitis relapse even months after survival of the Ebola disease (Jacobs et al., 2016). As the Ebola virus also persists in corpses, safe burials must be organized, and washing and touching of the deceased persons, as traditionally performed in the epidemic regions, must not be done (Lindblade et al., 2016).

For diagnosis of the Ebola disease, patients with typical symptoms should undergo rapid laboratory testing in order to confirm or rule out the presence of the Ebola virus. Frequent other diseases with fever, e.g., malaria or bacterial gastroenteritis, should be checked for and treated. During the diagnostic procedures, potentially infectious patients must be strictly isolated until they are proven to be free of the Ebola virus. Laboratory testing for the Ebola disease is mainly based on the detection of the viral genome by RT-PCR, providing reliable results from day three to symptoms onset. The RT-PCR method is however technically demanding and was unavailable at local points of care at the beginning of the outbreak (Butler, 2014).

Treatment options were largely limited to supportive care owing to the absence of approved of curative drugs. The mainstay of basic supportive care constitutes intravenous fluid and salt replacement therapy (Lamontagne et al., 2014), administrating up to 10 l per day per patient. The Ebola disease often affects multiple organs in its course, requiring extensive supportive care, including intensive care units equipped for ventilation or dialysis (Beeching et al., 2014). Such comprehensive supportive care is difficult to offer at the remote sites where the epidemic was spreading, and challenging to provide under conditions of patients' isolation. Maintaining supportive care for isolated cases requires extensive logistic support. Even under the best supportive care conditions in highly developed health care systems outside the epidemic area, deaths of patients were unavoidable owing to the lack of curative drugs. Out of 27 patients treated in US and European hospitals from August 2014 to December 2015, five patients died, resulting in a much lower mortality of 18.5 percent under the best supportive care conditions, compared to a mortality of up to 75 percent in some parts of the epidemic area (Uyeki et al., 2016). Of the patients treated in US and European hospitals, 22 were health care workers repatriated from the epidemic area. This low number of infected expatriate health care workers could hint at a rather low, but not absent infection risk under optimal precaution measures. Some of these patients became minutely documented in the medical literature and provided deeper insights into the disease course under optimal treatment conditions (Gulland, 2015; Yacisin et al., 2015). In contrast, a very high number of local health care workers were infected in the first year of the epidemic, with the WHO reporting 838 infected health care workers in January 2015, of whom 495, thus more than half, had died (Fox, 2015).

In parallel to the spreading of the Ebola disease in 2014, research on curative drugs for the Ebola disease were significantly increased. In the later phase of the epidemic, first, still unapproved, drugs became available in sparse amounts for clinical trials and questionable compassionate use (Lanini et al., 2015; PREVAIL II Writing Group, 2016). Furthermore, preventive vaccines are just being developed (Agnandji et al., 2016; Keshwara et al., 2017). These tools may help to prevent another Ebola epidemic of this magnitude in the future.

The 2014–16 Ebola outbreak has been a dramatic challenge to the affected populations and countries, the WHO, and the humanitarian and military personnel engaged in the fight against the spreading of the disease. While this contribution seeks to address the specific military medical ethics aspects that have been arising during these missions, the socioeconomic recovery in the affected countries is only at its beginning (Gostin and Friedman, 2015; Green, 2016; McBain et al., 2016).

Common ethical issues encountered during epidemics

Before presenting the outline and the chapters of the present volume, we want to give a brief and general overview of the ethical issues that often arise in the context of epidemics and that have been discussed in the literature. In doing so, we want to sketch the scene and provide the context against which the discussion in this volume takes place. While many of the ethical issues associated with epidemics are similar to those encountered in "ordinary" public health problems, the context of epidemics adds a layer to the complexity. To name a few examples, ethical issues arise around questions of restricting individual liberties when using patient isolation or large-scale quarantine measures to control the outbreak; allocation, domestic and international, of possibly scarce resources; the question of a duty to treat and the duty not to infect others; and the use of experimental treatment and doing research in disaster settings like epidemic areas. In the following pages, we want to introduce some of these ethical challenges. Obviously, this short section can only aim to roughly outline the issues and does not pretend to cover them in any extensive way.

Restricting individual liberties

Among the typical measures to control epidemics of infectious diseases are patient isolation and quarantine measures. Both measures are taken in order to prevent the spread of a disease and do not constitute therapeutic interventions to cure individual patients. Whereas isolation is used for patients who are symptomatic of the disease (which does not necessarily mean that they are diagnosed positive in the end), quarantine measures also apply to populations that are still asymptomatic but may have been previously exposed to carriers of the disease or may be deemed too untrustworthy to restrict themselves. Different ways of implementing different kinds of isolation or quarantine exist (ranging from high-security facility isolation to home-based quarantine) but all basically share the ethical issue of restricting individual liberties such as the freedom of movement or other basic (human) rights but also patients' autonomy. Justifications for such measures refer to the protection of a larger number of other people and thus weigh individual rights versus a collective good. In the context of international missions and when large numbers of people are affected by quarantine measures, the question by whom and how such measures should be enforced also becomes relevant. In this book, quarantine and isolation measures and some of the associated ethical issues will be discussed by several authors (mainly in Chapters 3, 6, 7, and 8).

Resource scarcity and just allocation

As epidemics by definition mean that a much larger number of people are affected by a disease than is usual, resources will sooner or later become scarce as emergency and disaster preparedness measures are exhausted. The just distribution of scarce and potentially life-saving resources poses another important and constant ethical challenge during epidemics. Resources, in this context, do not necessarily and exclusively consist of medication or technical equipment, but can also be health care personnel and even time that is spent per patient. The availability of sufficient resources is on the one hand a question of foresight and planning: disaster preparedness must weigh the costs of stocking etc. against risk and utility from a long-term perspective. In acute phases during the reaction to epidemics, the more pressing question is that of how and according to which criteria scarce resources shall be distributed. Here, much depends on the preparation, on whether an epidemic was expected, on whether the disease in question can be healed, and on what kind of resources are needed. As the case may be, missing resources may be replaced by fast reaction or improvization, or may result in ethical problems such as the need to triage patients.

As a result of a lack or scarcity of resources, we can often observe a lowering of the standards of care as more people than usual need to share the same amount of resources (levelling down effect). Such compromising of usual standards leads to situations that are clearly less than ideal: lower standards of medical care (with all related consequences for the patients) on the one hand and stress for health care providers (who feel that one could do better and who are on a higher workload) on the other hand come as inevitable consequences. In such situations, much depends on the questions of what are the (good?) reasons for the current (and lower) standards of care and whether they can be explained and are comprehensible. The Ebola epidemic has been an extremely strong challenge for these kinds of questions as, first, it occurred in countries with already low standards of medical care and scarce resources; second, the treatment of the disease needs lots of different resources; and, third, because the international response teams were used to quite different standards in their countries than during their emergency relief missions. In the present volume, the field reports provided in the first six chapters all discuss issues related to scarce resources to some extent.

Duty to treat

It is often assumed that professional health care workers have a duty to treat patients, even if this means that they may be exposed to personal risk. Numerous grounds have been offered for this view, including expressed consent, implied consent, special training, reciprocity, and professional oaths and codes. During epidemics with infectious diseases, the question of a "duty to treat" becomes especially important as the dangers involved in the treatment of infected persons are greater than usual and also become more obvious. In such contexts, it is thus argued that, when the risks are very high and the treatment benefits low, the duty to treat is significantly diminished; it then becomes less than categorical and may even be considered a supererogatory duty in extreme circumstances. Within the framework of this book, the question of a duty to care is taken up in more detail by the last two chapters, which both analyze arguments for a duty to care and add the second layer to what extent this duty is influenced by the adherence to the military profession. The latter is even more relevant in the context of epidemics as military health care personnel are often involved in the reaction to epidemics, be it domestically or (as in the recent Ebola outbreak) even in regions far from their home countries.

Research, experimental treatment, compassionate use

The question of research or the use of experimental treatments is not automatically connected to epidemics, but may arise when no (standard) medication or no gold standard of care is known for the disease. This is still the case for the Ebola disease, which, in addition, has a very high mortality rate. The combination of these two factors seems to have facilitated the acceptance of unproven medical interventions like compassionate use or off-label use of medications. Such emergency use of unproven interventions may well amount to research and should thus be subject to the ethical criteria and requirements that usually apply, like the Declaration of Helsinki. However, the environment or even disaster context during epidemics is very often not optimal for doing research to say the least. Usual criteria for doing research (like the necessity for informed consent, double blind study design, etc.) may be disrespected owing to the environment, the urgency, or the available resources. Even if done with good intentions, such an approach poses a lot of concerns and is ethically highly questionable. In this volume, the research aspect is not a central topic as it falls outside the scope of the issues encountered by military health care personnel in the Ebola epidemic, who are instead involved in emergency relief.

After this cursory overview of some of the most relevant ethical challenges posed by epidemics of infectious diseases, we will now introduce the chapters of this volume, illustrate how they relate to each other, and show how they cover different aspects and approaches to the main subject of the book: ethical challenges for military health care personnel faced with epidemics.

The chapters and their "common story"

The different chapters of this book offer insights into recent experiences from military and NGO missions during the 2014/15 Ebola outbreak in West Africa but also theoretical reflections on more general ethical subjects related to epidemics. The book, in a rather novel manner, combines the experience and reflections from an international group of authors with an interdisciplinary approach as the topics of the different chapters range from experience reports of military doctors to policy analyses and ethical reflections of academic philosophers. In doing so it aims at giving a voice to both the experiences from the ground (the "real world") and the reflection from academic distance (the "ivory tower"). We assume that the exchange between these two worlds can be fruitful, interesting, and relevant for both sides – even though at first sight they may not always understand or even appreciate each other.

The first four chapters of this volume offer insights into the planning of and the actual implementation of military medical relief missions of four nations (Canada, Germany, Russia, the United Kingdom) that were deployed to three different countries (the Republic of Guinea, Liberia, Sierra Leone) during the Ebola disease outbreak in 2014/15. The authors of these chapters can all base their reports on personal experience or on interviews conducted with deployed personnel and thus offer first-hand insights into the reality of those missions and the problems encountered.

In the opening chapter, Heather Draper and colleagues present and analyze interviews that have been conducted with British military medical staff (doctors, nurses, and other allied health care professionals) who were involved in the planning of the British mission to Sierra Leone during the 2014/15 Ebola outbreak. This chapter thus gives a direct insight into the experiences with the rather unusual mission that the military had to plan and enriches the interview findings with thorough academic analysis. The ethical issues reported by the interviewees ranged from very general considerations at the beginning of the planning, when the whole mission was questioned, to questions about who and should be selected for treatment and per what rules, and rather specific issues such as the use of surveillance cameras and their possible interference with patients' privacy. The chapter also discusses the duties of the state vis-à-vis to the deployed personnel and discusses the question of their preferred treatment if they get infected and the question of their possible repatriation as patients.

Another focus of the authors' research is about the preparation of training material for future similar missions. During the interviews, the questions were also asked to what extent the participants felt prepared to meet the ethical challenges on the ground, what resources they drew on to meet them, and what additional training and support they would recommend to/for others prior to similar deployment. The last section of the present chapter presents a first sample of the training material that is going to be developed on the basis of the experiences during the Sierra Leone mission.

Ivan Kholikov and Kira Sazonova in the first part of their chapter report the problems and challenges associated with the deployment of the material for a Russian field hospital to the Republic of Guinea and in the second part offer some legal reflections. Their field report tells the sometimes very practical problems encountered during the transfer and setting up of a field hospital and illustrates the complicated nature of a seemingly rather simple mission. Kholikov, who was the leader of the Russian team, walks the reader through the considerable amount of various organizational, ethical, and legal challenges that the Russian team faced during their mission. Among these obstacles were local authorities unwilling to cooperate, false information around the Ebola disease in general, and issues of using experimental treatment and quarantine encountered by the deployed personnel, especially on their way back to Russia. In the second part of their chapter, the authors provide some thoughts on how to approach epidemic outbreaks from an international law perspective. More precisely, they analyse the notion of international responsibility and show how it can be used to justify state obligations to prevent the proliferation of diseases and, thus, epidemics. The relevance of the international legal perspective is underlined by the fact that the UN Security Council declared the 2014 Ebola outbreak a "threat to international peace and security" in its Resolution 2177(2014). The authors conclude, however, that the idea of international responsibility only starts to become applied in contexts of epidemics and infectious diseases.

Christian Janke's chapter is based on field experience of the author as a doctor in a German Ebola treatment unit deployed to Liberia. Janke's analysis is based on the problems encountered during the mission in 2015, a mission that took quite some time until the deployment and eventually came close to no longer being needed. The chapter focuses on the management and mismanagement of (suspected) Ebola cases and the problem of cross-infection in treatment facilities. The chapter treats some ethical aspects related to the question of how patients with Ebola-like symptoms have been selected and cared for by international responders. Most importantly, it is concerned with showing how different categories of suspected cases must be treated differently and should be separated from each other in order to avoid a spread of the infectious disease to noninfected patients who only exhibit similar symptoms. On a more theoretical level, the chapter reads the conflict between adequately caring for individuals and doing the best for all as a conflict between human rights and utilitarian ethics. Crisis management, according to the authors, has to consider at least some utilitarian thinking to be successful.

Paul Eagan analyzes the domestic and international reaction of the Canadian government to the Ebola outbreak and specifically focuses on the role attributed to and played by the Canadian Armed Forces. The author was involved in formulating and delivering the Canadian Armed Forces' response to the Ebola epidemic and at the time, served as head of the communicable disease control section and was acting director of the Directorate of Force Health Protection of the Canadian Armed Forces. Eagan's chapter includes an overview and analysis of the ethical issues that informed Canadian policy decisions in reaction to the 2014/15 Ebola outbreak. Among the ethical issues that were anticipated or encountered are the role of the military as a provider of humanitarian assistance, the question of how to allocate scarce medical resources, the use of experimental vaccines in situations such as epidemics, and the question of how to use quarantine measures. The chapter ends in asserting that most of the ethical issues were not specific to Ebola but could also be encountered in the context of different epidemics. Consequently, it is important to keep the lessons learned in the past and try to avoid repeating them in the future.

Chapters 5 and 6 of this volume are also both chapters that are widely informed by experiences on the ground. They however slightly change the perspective and look at the pressures and the moral burden put on both (military) health care personnel and Ebola victims during the outbreak of the epidemic.

The study presented by Jill Horning and colleagues amends former work during which four sources of ethical challenge for military and humanitarian health care workers were identified: first, resource scarcity; second, historical, cultural, or social structures; third, existing policies and regulations; and, fourth, professional roles and their associated obligations. Even though the data on which the chapter is based is taken from a different mission and context, the findings are still relevant for the context of humanitarian relief missions. The 2014/15 Ebola outbreak, with its context of a disease-related "mass casualty situation" (without combat and conflict), offers new dimensions of the well-known ethical challenges such as voluntariness and motivations for deployment, willingness to work with uncertainty, and the exigencies of research and public health contexts on clinical experience of health workers. The chapter offers an analysis of these new problems and an overview of factors that influence or can cause moral distress among health care personnel.

From the perspective and experience of humanitarian workers (within Médecins Sans Frontières, MSF), Philippe Calain and Marc Poncin look at the recent Ebola crisis as another testing moment for public health ethics as it is exposing new dimensions of the tension between individual or patient autonomy and the common good. The authors shed light at often-used but nevertheless unpopular measures, such as home quarantine, travel restrictions, the forcible isolation of possible cases, or periods of lockdown that create ethically difficult situations. For (civilian) health workers, and particularly for outreach teams, these measures make it difficult to avoid being assimilated with law enforcement authorities. For victims and their families, facility isolation after Ebola contamination is on the other hand probably the most onerous of all recognized public health measures. Thus, contact tracers and case finders are often facing difficult dilemmas, when public health actions to limit contagion conflict with the obligation to respect the patients' autonomy and their human dignity. The authors warn that limits between persuasion, coercion, and deception are difficult to draw in situations where facility isolation essentially equals to a self-sacrifice of the patients. The moral burden put by these measures both on health care workers but also on Ebola victims is a different face of public health measures that has not received much attention so far.

The last four chapters offer more theoretical analyses and philosophical reflections on two of the most pressing ethical issues encountered during outbreaks of epidemics, namely the use of quarantine or isolation to fight against communicable diseases and second the question to what extent health care personnel should fulfil what is called a "moral duty to care."

In Chapter 7, Cécile Bensimon and Ana Komparic give an overview of the history and development of quarantine both from a theoretical perspective and regarding historical examples. They conceptualize their narrative of the development of quarantine around the conflict between individual (liberty) rights on the one hand and public health on the other hand. Quarantine is among the oldest measures to control the infiltration of communicable diseases into local communities and to fight against epidemics. Nevertheless, the contemporary criticism of its use based on its negative impact on individual rights is relatively new and can be tied to the development and institutionalization of human rights. This is illustrated in the chapter on the debate of how to control communicable diseases in the context of the emergence of the HIV/AIDS epidemic. The historical overview also serves as a basis to contextualize the issues raised about the use of quarantine during the 2014/15 Ebola outbreak and to explain why quarantine remains a both important and contentious means in the tool kit of public health measures.

Sheena M. Eagan gives a contemporary exemplum of the use of quarantine and analyzes one specific public health measure of the US government following the recent Ebola outbreak, namely the controversial 21-day quarantine plan issued in October 2014 for American service members returning from areas in West Africa affected by Ebola virus outbreaks. More specifically, she looks at the ethical issues involved in the American policy of what has been called "controlled monitoring," or quarantine, in the US armed forces. Among these issues are the questions whether this policy represented an excessive infringement on autonomy and individual rights, or whether it was a necessary measure in disease control. Eagan evaluates the US policy by applying a framework of public health ethics, but she also considers some uniquely military factors, including the complicated questions regarding the limited autonomy of soldiers, and the related obligations of the military institution and military command. Her chapter thus amends the previous historical chapter and illustrates the ongoing relevance of ethical issues related to quarantine.

In a theoretical chapter, Daniel Messelken looks at the philosophical question of whether and to what extent doctors and other health care personnel can legitimately be said to have a moral duty to care even if, for example during epidemics, this may imperil their own health. The chapter gives a review of the philosophical literature on the duty to care and the question of imposed risk-taking by medical personnel. Messelken then extends the discussion to include the question of the extent to which military medical personnel can be justifiably expected to act according to these duties in the same way as their civilian counterparts or whether military health care personnel might act under a different moral obligation – with more or less encompassing or at least different duties. The chapter thus addresses both the general question of a moral basis for a duty to care in general and the more precise issue of a duty of military medical personnel to provide such care during epidemics in distant countries.

In a similar way to the preceding chapter, Paul Gilbert raises the question of how drafting military physicians to engage in humanitarian missions to assist Ebola-affected countries can be justified from a moral perspective. He starts from the assumption that it is ethically unclear to what extent military doctors can be expected to risk their own well-being outside their usual duties of keeping members of the armed forces fit for service and treating the casualties of combat. After a review of different scenarios in which military doctors may be confronted with epidemics, Gilbert considers two potential types of justification for their being required to assist in treating the victims of epidemics like Ebola: first, that this medical assistance is a form of humanitarian intervention; second, that it is analogous to military actions of self-defence in helping to prevent harm to one's own population. Both arguments can be referred to in order to justify the drafting or military doctors but both also set limits to how far such drafting can go.

Outlook

As we write this introduction, the Ebola epidemic in West Africa has come to an end and its spread to a pandemic in the larger region or on a global scale was fortunately prevented. Unfortunately, other epidemics of Ebola or similarly deadly diseases will occur in the future and will make concerted responses necessary. It is therefore key to prepare for such kinds of events, on the one hand, on the technical and logistical level, to be able to rapidly react and deploy appropriate means and personnel and, on the other hand, on a more abstract level, for the ethical challenges that epidemics and the associated missions will (again) generate in the future. This volume wants to contribute to the latter by analyzing what has happened and which challenges have been successfully met. Besides planning and imagination, it is learning from experience that can help us avoid falling into the same traps as before.

Notes

1 www.who.int/topics/infectious_diseases/en (accessed October 9, 2016).
2 www.who.int/hac/about/definitions/en/, our italics (accessed October 9, 2016).
3 www.afro.who.int/en/clusters-a-programmes/dpc/epidemic-a-pandemic-alert-and-response/4065-ebola-virus-disease-in-guinea-25-march-2014.html (accessed October 9, 2016).
4 www.who.int/mediacentre/news/statements/2014/ebola-20140808/en (accessed October 9, 2016).
5 All statistics in this paragraph are taken from the CDC's infographics, which are available online at www.cdc.gov/vhf/ebola/pdf/cost-ebola-multipage-infographic.pdf.

A general overview by the CDC is available online at www.cdc.gov/vhf/ebola/outbreaks/2014-west-africa/cost-of-ebola.html (both pages accessed October 9, 2016).

6 www.ifrc.org/en/what-we-do/disaster-management/about-disasters (accessed October 9, 2016).

7 During the 2014–16 epidemic, MSF treated one-third of all Ebola virus disease patients in their facilities. See www.msf.org/en/article/report-ebola-2014–2015-facts-figures (accessed October 9, 2016).

References

Agnandji, S. T., Huttner, A., Zinser, M. E., Njuguna, P., Dahlke, C., Fernandes, J. F., Yerly, S., Dayer, J. A., Kraehling, V., Kasonta, R., Adegnika, A. A., Altfeld, M., Auderset, F., Bache, E. B., Biedenkopf, N., Borregaard, S., Brosnahan, J. S., Burrow, R., Combescure, C., Desmeules, J., Eickmann, M., Fehling, S. K., Finckh, A., Goncalves, A. R., Grobusch, M. P., Hooper, J., Jambrecina, A., Kabwende, A. L., Kaya, G., Kimani, D., Lell, B., Lemaitre, B., Lohse, A. W., Massinga-Loembe, M., Matthey, A., Mordmuller, B., Nolting, A., Ogwang, C., Ramharter, M., Schmidt-Chanasit, J., Schmiedel, S., Silvera, P., Stahl, F. R., Staines, H. M., Strecker, T., Stubbe, H. C., Tsofa, B., Zaki, S., Fast, P., Moorthy, V., Kaiser, L., Krishna, S., Becker, S., Kieny, M. P., Bejon, P., Kremsner, P. G., Addo, M. M. and Siegrist, C. A. 2016. Phase 1 trials of rVSV Ebola vaccine in Africa and Europe. *New England Journal of Medicine*, 374, 1647–1660.

Baize, S., Pannetier, D., Oestereich, L., Rieger, T., Koivogui, L., Magassouba, N. F., Soropogui, B., Sow, M. S., Keïta, S., De Clerck, H., Tiffany, A., Dominguez, G., Loua, M., Traoré, A., Kolié, M., Malano, E. R., Heleze, E., Bocquin, A., Mély, S., Raoul, H., Caro, V., Cadar, D., Gabriel, M., Pahlmann, M., Tappe, D., Schmidt-Chanasit, J., Impouma, B., Diallo, A. K., Formenty, P., Van Herp, M. and Günther, S. 2014. Emergence of Zaire Ebola virus disease in Guinea. *New England Journal of Medicine*, 371, 1418–1425.

Bausch, D. G., Nichol, S. T., Muyembe-Tamfum, J. J., Borchert, M., Rollin, P. E., Sleurs, H., Campbell, P., Tshioko, F. K., Roth, C., Colebunders, R., Pirard, P., Mardel, S., Olinda, L. A., Zeller, H., Tshomba, A., Kulidri, A., Libande, M. L., Mulangu, S., Formenty, P., Grein, T., Leirs, H., Braack, L., Ksiazek, T., Zaki, S., Bowen, M. D., Smit, S. B., Leman, P. A., Burt, F. J., Kemp, A., Swanepoel, R. and International Scientific and Technical Committee for Marburg Hemorrhagic Fever Control in the Democratic Republic of the Congo. 2006. Marburg hemorrhagic fever associated with multiple genetic lineages of virus. *New England Journal of Medicine*, 355, 909–919.

Beeching, N. J., Fenech, M. and Houlihan, C. F. 2014. Ebola virus disease. *BMJ*, 349, g7348.

Burki, T. K. 2016. Post-Ebola syndrome. *Lancet Infectious Diseases*, 16, 780–781.

Butler, D. 2014. Ebola experts seek to expand testing. *Nature*, 516, 154–155.

Chertow, D. S., Kleine, C., Edwards, J. K., Scaini, R., Giuliani, R. and Sprecher, A. 2014. Ebola virus disease in West Africa–clinical manifestations and management. *New England Journal of Medicine*, 371, 2054–2057.

Fowler, R., Mishra, S. and Chan, A. K. 2016. The crucial importance of long-term follow-up for Ebola virus survivors. *Lancet Infectious Diseases*, 16, 987–989.

Fox, M. 2015. *Ebola Kills Nearly 500 Health Care Workers*. NBC News.

Gostin, L. O. and Friedman, E. A. 2015. A retrospective and prospective analysis of the west African Ebola virus disease epidemic: robust national health systems at the foundation and an empowered WHO at the apex. *Lancet*, 385, 1902–1909.

Green, A. 2016. West African countries focus on post-Ebola recovery plans. *Lancet*, 388, 2463–2465.

Gulland, A. 2015. Nurse with Ebola virus remains in critical condition. *BMJ*, 350, h36.

Heymann, D. L., Chen, L., Takemi, K., Fidler, D. P., Tappero, J. W., Thomas, M. J., Kenyon, T. A., Frieden, T. R., Yach, D., Nishtar, S., Kalache, A., Olliaro, P. L., Horby, P., Torreele, E., Gostin, L. O., Ndomondo-Sigonda, M., Carpenter, D., Rushton, S., Lillywhite, L., Devkota, B., Koser, K., Yates, R., Dhillon, R. S. and Rannan-Eliya, R. P. 2015. Global health security: the wider lessons from the West African Ebola virus disease epidemic. *Lancet*, 385, 1884–1901.

International Commission. 1978. Ebola haemorrhagic fever in Zaire, 1976. *Bulletin of the World Health Organization*, 56, 271–293.

Jacobs, M., Rodger, A., Bell, D. J., Bhagani, S., Cropley, I., Filipe, A., Gifford, R. J., Hopkins, S., Hughes, J., Jabeen, F., Johannessen, I., Karageorgopoulos, D., Lackenby, A., Lester, R., Liu, R. S., MacConnachie, A., Mahungu, T., Martin, D., Marshall, N., Mepham, S., Orton, R., Palmarini, M., Patel, M., Perry, C., Peters, S. E., Porter, D., Ritchie, D., Ritchie, N. D., Seaton, R. A., Sreenu, V. B., Templeton, K., Warren, S., Wilkie, G. S., Zambon, M., Gopal, R. and Thomson, E. C. 2016. Late Ebola virus relapse causing meningoencephalitis: a case report. *Lancet*, 388, 498–503.

Keshwara, R., Johnson, R. F. and Schnell, M. J. 2017. Toward an effective Ebola virus vaccine. *Annual Review of Medicine*, 68, 371–386.

Lamontagne, F., Clement, C., Fletcher, T., Jacob, S. T., Fischer, W. A., 2nd and Fowler, R. A. 2014. Doing today's work superbly well – treating Ebola with current tools. *New England Journal of Medicine*, 371, 1565–1566.

Lanini, S., Zumla, A., Ioannidis, J. P., Di Caro, A., Krishna, S., Gostin, L., Girardi, E., Pletschette, M., Strada, G., Baritussio, A., Portella, G., Apolone, G., Cavuto, S., Satolli, R., Kremsner, P., Vairo, F. and Ippolito, G. 2015. Are adaptive randomised trials or non-randomised studies the best way to address the Ebola outbreak in west Africa? *Lancet Infectious Diseases*, 15, 738–745.

Lindblade, K. A., Nyenswah, T., Keita, S., Diallo, B., Kateh, F., Amoah, A., Nagbe, T. K., Raghunathan, P., Neatherlin, J. C., Kinzer, M., Pillai, S. K., Attfield, K. R., Hajjeh, R., Dweh, E., Painter, J., Barradas, D. T., Williams, S. G., Blackley, D. J., Kirking, H. L., Patel, M. R., Dea, M., Massoudi, M. S., Barskey, A. E., Zarecki, S. L., Fomba, M., Grube, S., Belcher, L., Broyles, L. N., Maxwell, T. N., Hagan, J. E., Yeoman, K., Westercamp, M., Mott, J., Mahoney, F., Slutsker, L., DeCock, K. M., Marston, B. and Dahl, B. 2016. Secondary infections with Ebola virus in rural communities, Liberia and Guinea, 2014–2015. *Emerging Infectious Diseases*, 22, 1653–1655.

Mate, S. E., Kugelman, J. R., Nyenswah, T. G., Ladner, J. T., Wiley, M. R., Cordier-Lassalle, T., Christie, A., Schroth, G. P., Gross, S. M., Davies-Wayne, G. J., Shinde, S. A., Murugan, R., Sieh, S. B., Badio, M., Fakoli, L., Taweh, F., de Wit, E., van Doremalen, N., Munster, V. J., Pettitt, J., Prieto, K., Humrighouse, B. W., Stroher, U., DiClaro, J. W., Hensley, L. E., Schoepp, R. J., Safronetz, D., Fair, J., Kuhn, J. H., Blackley, D. J., Laney, A. S., Williams, D. E., Lo, T., Gasasira, A., Nichol, S. T., Formenty, P., Kateh, F. N., DeCock, K. M., Bolay, F., Sanchez-Lockhart, M. and Palacios, G. 2015. Molecular evidence of sexual transmission of Ebola virus. *New England Journal of Medicine*, 373, 2448–2454.

McBain, R. K., Wickett, E., Mugunga, J. C., Beste, J., Konwloh, P. and Mukherjee, J. 2016. The post-Ebola baby boom: time to strengthen health systems. *Lancet*, 388, 2331–2333.

McCloskey, B., Dar, O., Zumla, A. and Heymann, D. L. 2014. Emerging infectious diseases and pandemic potential: status quo and reducing risk of global spread. *Lancet Infectious Diseases*, 14, 1001–1010.

Médecins Sans Frontières. 2015. *Pushed to the Limit and Beyond. A Year into the Largest Ever Ebola Outbreak.* Geneva: Médecins Sans Frontières.

Meltzer, M. I., Atkins, C. Y., Santibanez, S., Knust, B., Petersen, B. W., Ervin, E. D., Nichol, S. T., Damon, I. K. and Washington, M. L. 2014. Estimating the future number of cases in the Ebola epidemic – Liberia and Sierra Leone, 2014–2015. *Morbidity and Mortality Weekly Report Supplement*, 63, 1–14.

Porta, M. S. 2014. *A Dictionary of Epidemiology*. Oxford, Oxford University Press.

PREVAIL II Writing Group. 2016. A randomized, controlled trial of ZMapp for Ebola virus infection. *New England Journal of Medicine*, 375, 1448–1456.

Sands, P., Mundaca-Shah, C. and Dzau, V. J. 2016. The neglected dimension of global security – a framework for countering infectious-disease crises. *New England Journal of Medicine*, 374, 1281–1287.

Team, W. H. O. E. R. 2014. Ebola virus disease in West Africa – the first 9 months of the epidemic and forward projections. *New England Journal of Medicine*, 371, 1481–1495.

Urbanowicz, R. A., McClure, C. P., Sakuntabhai, A., Sall, A. A., Kobinger, G., Muller, M. A., Holmes, E. C., Rey, F. A., Simon-Loriere, E. and Ball, J. K. 2016. Human adaptation of Ebola virus during the West African Outbreak. *Cell*, 167, 1079–1087, e5.

Uyeki, T. M., Mehta, A. K., Davey, R. T., Jr., Liddell, A. M., Wolf, T., Vetter, P., Schmiedel, S., Grunewald, T., Jacobs, M., Arribas, J. R., Evans, L., Hewlett, A. L., Brantsaeter, A. B., Ippolito, G., Rapp, C., Hoepelman, A. I. and Gutman, J., for the Working Group of the, U.S.–European Clinical Network on Clinical Management of Ebola Virus Disease Patients in the U.S. and Europe. 2016. Clinical management of Ebola virus disease in the United States and Europe. *New England Journal of Medicine*, 374, 636–646.

Varkey, J. B., Shantha, J. G., Crozier, I., Kraft, C. S., Lyon, G. M., Mehta, A. K., Kumar, G., Smith, J. R., Kainulainen, M. H., Whitmer, S., Stroher, U., Uyeki, T. M., Ribner, B. S. and Yeh, S. 2015. Persistence of Ebola virus in ocular fluid during convalescence. *New England Journal of Medicine*, 372, 2423–2427.

Vetter, P., Fischer, W. A., 2nd, Schibler, M., Jacobs, M., Bausch, D. G. and Kaiser, L. 2016. Ebola virus shedding and transmission: review of current evidence. *Journal of Infectious Diseases*, 214, S177–S184.

WHO. 2016. *Ebola Virus Disease Situation Report 10 June 2016*. Geneva: WHO.

WHO/International Study Team 1978. Ebola haemorrhagic fever in Sudan, 1976. Report of a WHO/International Study Team. *Bulletin of the World Health Organization*, 56, 247–270.

Yacisin, K., Balter, S., Fine, A., Weiss, D., Ackelsberg, J., Prezant, D., Wilson, R., Starr, D., Rakeman, J., Raphael, M., Quinn, C., Toprani, A., Clark, N., Link, N., Daskalakis, D., Maybank, A., Layton, M. and Varma, J. K., for the Centers for Disease Control & Prevention. 2015. Ebola virus disease in a humanitarian aid worker – New York City, October 2014. *Morbidity and Mortality Weekly Report*, 64, 321–323.

Zumla, A., Hui, D. S. and Perlman, S. 2015. Middle East respiratory syndrome. *Lancet*, 386, 995–1007.

1 Preparing for Operation GRITROCK

Military medical ethics challenges encountered in the planning stages of the UK Ebola response mission

Heather Draper, Simon Jenkins, Lizzy Bernthal, Catherine Hale, Jeremy Henning and Chris Gibson

Introduction

In early September 2014, Médecins Sans Frontières (MSF) took the unusual step of calling on governments to deploy military, as well as civilian, assets to help combat the Ebola virus disease (EVD) epidemic raging in West Africa (MSF, 2014). The UK government announced a package of aid in response to the outbreak, including the deployment of military experts, targeted primarily on Sierra Leone (Gov.uk, 2014). The scale of the outbreak and the responses to it attracted comment from many quarters and raised ethical issues. We were interested in the ethical challenges that would confront the troops on the ground in Sierra Leone, particularly those who were health care professionals. We successfully secured UK funding council research funds to explore these challenges. During the preparatory stages of this project, however, it became clear that ethical decisions had also been made during the planning stages of the deployment in anticipation of issue that may be faced on the deployment. These planning issues are of interest in their own right, even though they fell outside the aims of our project, and we explore of some these in this chapter.

We will start with a brief background to the British medical military involvement in Sierra Leone during the 2014–15 EBV outbreak in West Africa. We then outline and discuss some of the ethical challenges that confronted those involved in the planning for the military side of this operation. As one of our aims was to use the experiences of those who deployed to produce materials that could be used in future ethics training for both military and civilian humanitarian responders going forward, we have included an example based around one of the issues explored in this chapter, namely whether it is permissible to use surveillance cameras in an Ebola treatment unit.

Background

Operation GRITROCK was the name given to the British Ministry of Defence (MOD) mission in Sierra Leone during the 2014–15 EVD outbreak.[1] Among other measures, military clinical and clinical support staff were deployed in two distinct kinds of role: to provide general, non-EVD-related health care support for deployed military and other eligible personnel, and to staff a small EVD treatment unit (ETU) for EVD-affected health care workers and other eligible personnel. This chapter will focus on preparations in relation to the latter role.

It is fair to say that the UK Defence Medical Service (DMS) had less recent experience in purely humanitarian response than other national military services.[2] The main focus of DMS over preceding years had been on supporting UK troops in Afghanistan. Most DMS personnel with any deployment experience had deployed at least once to the Role Three hospital in Camp Bastion. With the withdrawal of British forces planned for October 2014, however, DMS had at the time of the EVD outbreak in West Africa already moved to contingency training/planning. Potential deployment as part of a UK government response to a humanitarian disaster or emergency had already been anticipated, though perhaps with more of a focus on trauma care than an infectious disease outbreak. Indeed, the UK government strategic defence and security review, published in November 2015 (HM Government, 2015), places humanitarian assistance first on the list of available responses:

> The Armed Forces will also contribute to the Government's response to crises by being prepared to:

> - Support humanitarian assistance and disaster response, and conduct rescue missions.
> - Conduct strike operations.
> - Conduct operations to restore peace and stability.
> - Conduct major combat operations if required, including under NATO Article 5.

Moreover, the threat to national and global security by emergent microbial disease is also highlighted in the review. Accordingly, we should expect that the British medical military will have an increasing humanitarian response role going forward.

Responding quickly to the EVD outbreak was a considerable challenge that required innovation in terms of training and protocols and was beyond the existing experience of many of those involved. Moreover, the military deployment was part of a cross-governmental response that involved the Department for International Development (DFID), Foreign Office and Department of Health, among others. As Bricknell *et al.* (2015) noted,

> There was an early acknowledgement that there should be a strong medical voice as part of the military-planning process as this was a public health crisis rather than the usual DMS role of providing medical support to a military plan.

> (Bricknell *et al.*, 2015, p. 170)

Moreover, any plans had to take into account that the MOD

> had responsibilities as an employer to ensure that any risks to health and safety [of military personnel ordered to deploy] were fully assessed, mitigated and any residual risk managed to be as low as reasonably practicable.
>
> (Bricknell *et al.*, 2015, p. 170)

Furthermore, DFID retained responsibility for purchasing equipment for the ETU. Finally, a general election had already been called for May 2015. It is reasonable to assume that any party in government, or any one of the opposition parties, would seek to gain maximum political capital from the national response to the EVD outbreak, and also to minimize any potential political damage as a consequence of this response. Thus, these sorts of political preoccupation may have influenced how the UK response in Africa was offered, funded and executed, but also – once the seriousness of the outbreak had been accepted – government plans for preventing or managing any spread to the UK, by whatever means that spread might occur.

One advantage that the British military had was that of prior experience in Sierra Leone. In spring 2000, British forces were deployed to evacuate foreign nationals during the civil war (Operation PALLISER), an operation that was expanded as evacuations plans were jeopardised when the Revolutionary United Front prevented access to Lungi airport. British military forces were involved in training the Sierra Leonean military, including restoring its medical military capability. The military operation, and more specifically the actions of the Commander British Forces General (Brigadier at the time) David Richards, are conjectured to have brought the civil war to an early end (Renton, 2010; Little, 2010; Richards, 2014). For this reason, the British military had a positive reputation in Sierra Leone. This, according to some of our informants, made it easier for troops in uniform to enter Sierra Leone without this being interpreted as a covert military combat intervention and generating local hostility. At the same time, the military was also well aware of how austere an environment Sierra Leone was to operate in, even without the threat of EVD. Historically, West Africa was dubbed the 'white man's grave' by Europeans (Curtin, 1990) because of the endemic cerebral malaria and yellow fever, among other things such as some of the most venomous snakes in the world. Of the population (aged 15–49 years) in 2014, 1.4 per cent was estimated to be infected with HIV (UNAIDS, 2014), which would need to be considered when deciding on the treatment package that should be available in the ETU, and sanitation infrastructure remains poor, especially in rural areas (UNICEF, 2015).

The international agreement covering military involvement in humanitarian relief (the Oslo Guidelines) states that military or civil defence assets can only be used as a 'last resort' in circumstances when there is 'no comparable civilian alternative' and when military assets would help bridge the 'humanitarian gap' and provide unique advantages in terms of capability, availability and timeliness, and would 'complement civilian capability' and 'meet a critical humanitarian need' (OCHA, 2007). Military humanitarian deployments are therefore only meant to be a short-term measure. Accordingly, the DMS was planning to staff the ETU for 60 days, before handing responsibility over to an NGO (Connor *et al.*, 2015). In the event, the responsibility for the unit was not relinquished until June 2015, and four consecutive cohorts of clinical and support staff were deployed.

Methodology

We designed a qualitative study to explore the challenges that military medical personnel faced during Operation GRITROCK, with a view to using this data to create training materials to assist deployees on similar future operations (see last section). To inform the interview guide for the main participant interviews, we conducted five preliminary interviews with key informants. We refer to these people as 'key informants' to distinguish them from 'participants' (those who later took part in the study itself). These key informant interviews were semi-structured and each lasted approximately one hour. Key informants were selected using purposive sampling. They were chosen on the basis of having played a central role in advising the UK government before the UK response was announced, and/or then having a central role in ensuring the success of the operation before it started, e.g. designing and delivering training to those deploying, collaborating on identifying equipment and writing standard operating procedures. Four had a clinical background and one did not. Four were in senior 'command' positions. The key informants understood the purpose of the interview and that it would be recorded. Written or verbal consent (audio-recorded) was also obtained. The interviews were transcribed for ease of access to the data and to ensure accuracy, but were not formally coded (unlike the participant interviews).

In addition, field notes were taken during observations of pre-deployment training being delivered to Canadian and British personnel at the Army Medical Services Field Training Centre (AMSTC), Strensall, UK. Notes were also taken of conversations with those running and assessing the training (with their knowledge and agreement) during this period of observation. Some of those not formally interviewed who provided information at this point later participated in the study. These field notes were used in combination with the main ethical issues identified by the key informants to develop the interview guide for the later, larger set of interviews. Some of these ethical issues are reported and explored in the following section. The ethical commentary on these issues reflects the views of the authors and not those of the key informants, the DMS or the MOD.

Some of the ethical issues

The ethical concerns around the decision to commit DMS personnel to treat EVD, eligibility criteria and risk were raised by more than one person. The issue of evacuation was raised in some form by everyone, and while the balance between informing troops and maintaining morale was mentioned by only one key informant, it was also described in the larger interview set (as a minor theme); the use of closed-circuit television (CCTV) cameras emerged during the field work in Strensall.

The planning for what became Operation GRITROCK started in July 2014 and the ETU was built and staffed ready to accept patients by the end of October 2014. In between was an intense period of activity including reconnaissance in September to determine whether it would be possible to set up treatment units and whether a unit should be set up and staffed by the DMS. Pre-deployment training also had to be devised and provided, based on simultaneous planning for how the ETU would run, with what equipment, and what level of service to provide. In addition, the reconnaissance had identified the need to assist the Sierra Leonean government in planning and coordinating the local crisis response, and to provide local workers with training in the use of personal pro-tective equipment (PPE), in which the military also played a prominent role. This took place against the backdrop of the outbreak intensifying in severity, with modelling over the summer months suggesting expediential increases in the numbers of those affected in the coming months (though this turned out to be mistaken (Butler, 2014)). In addition, there was increasing media interest at this time, and international debate on how best to contain the spread of infection. Over the summer of 2014, borders in neighbouring countries were intermittently closed, whole communities were 'locked down' and airlines suspended flights to affected areas.

'Making the call'

The interviews with key informants suggested that those charged with advising the government struggled with the ethical issues that surrounded deploying the military to have an active role in the care of those afflicted with the EVD virus. For instance, one prominent issue was whether this could be done effectively while simultaneously guaranteeing medical support for British troops elsewhere in the world, including combat troops should the need arise. Related to this, and given the estimates in circulation about the scale and duration of the outbreak, there was a need to have a clear exit strategy, which required there to be in place an identified organization to whom responsibility for the ETU could be handed. Clearly, this kind of consideration speaks to the prime organizational responsib-ility of the DMS and need not be debated further here. There were operational concerns about how few of the DMS staff were already trained to deal with infectious disease, and also concerns about an absence of existing kit, policies and procedures in a medical service that, up to this point, had been geared prim-arily towards treating trauma. Finally, there were concerns about how dangerous the mission would be, how effectively the risk to the troops could be mitigated and the degree of confidence there could be in the predicted risk calculations. In talking to our key informants, we found that individuals had different ways of evaluating these kinds of concerns. For one, the final justification rested on that individual's understanding of what the military was for:

> I equated it to a special forces uh hostage rescue mission, where we as a nation demonstrate that we will do everything we can in order to look after our people if they're in trouble ... some of our bravest and best as a nation ... had deployed out to that country for no reward financially, but only to try and help ... we should be proud of our nation's ability to produce people like that, and if they get into that situation then they should be supported.

For another, the justification seemed to be located more in the obligations that flowed from being a health care professional:

> there was a very strong ... moral push from the clinicians that we should be doing something and indeed also er that our heritage is very much in development of erm infectious disease ... so this this was a natural er thing for us to do.

Another spoke about being very concerned about the risks because:

> you can take interventions to reduce chances of something happening but the event, when it happens, is still catastrophic ... an individual may develop a severe infection and die... no matter what you could do, you're still going to be left with a significant risk [that] people become ill and die.

For this informant, the risk assessment appeared to be influenced by a strong sense of obligation to juniors: 'I was worried about the safety of my people and was I actually doing the right thing in endorsing it [the decision to deploy]'.

It was interesting for us to see, once all of the study data had been analysed, that this division between a military understanding of the mission and what we called a more humanitarian understanding of the mission was also found in how the participants themselves evaluated and understood the risks involved. This was also the case for the strong desire to protect those in their command, conceived as a military obligation owed to those commanded.

Determining the medical rules of eligibility (MRoE)

At the time that Operation GRITROCK was in the planning phase, predictions about the course of the outbreak were pretty dire (see above). Initial capability was sufficient only for a small, eight-bed ETU (with four beds for recovery, making 12 in total). This unit would be reserved for health care professionals (and other eligible persons). The ETU that was staffed by the British (and later Canadian) military was only part of the UK response. Other treatment units were built with the help of British military expertise, including a 70-bed unit – to be run by Save the Children, with funding support from DFID – that would cater for the general population.

The rationale for establishing a unit for health care professionals was described by our informants in the following terms:

> We were deploying a 12-bed Ebola treatment facility. Not to try and stop the spread of Ebola and treat everybody that deserved care, but to stiffen the resolve and confidence of overseas workers that were coming to the country to help. It was all about sustaining the will of healthcare workers to stag on.

This view is reflected in the account of the operation provided by Bricknell and colleagues:

> In the early stages of planning, the government's medical advice was to retain Ebola cases in country to reduce the risk of transmission in the UK. It was agreed that this would require the best available hospital services to be deployed *to provide reassurance to volunteers and their families that they would receive care at a standard comparable to that which would be delivered in the UK.*
>
> (Bricknell *et al.*, 2015, emphasis added)

Given that planners were anticipating arriving into a situation of huge need, it was decided that the beds in this unit would need to be strictly ring-fenced in order to maintain confidence.

> I thought that we would struggle to cope just with healthcare workers … that we would eventually have to turn healthcare workers away … there was significant pressure, understandably from the clinicians, to say why can't we take more people? … we should be filling up our beds with those in need … because they're good people and they want to be useful and want to help.… So that was a dilemma that I hadn't envisaged happening. Because I thought the beds would be full. But actually we had the ethical dilemma of empty beds in a Ebola treatment facility and people dying outside. But if I responded to the clinician's claim and said right fill the beds up with non-entitled but next week suddenly we get an outbreak in a Ebola hospital somewhere and we have ten international staff that needed a bed, and wouldn't be able to come in because we'd had the non-entitled there.

It was against this background that the MRoE were devised (and the empty beds referred to created, according to our participants, the most prevalent and difficult of the ethical challenges they faced on deployment). However, even at the planning phase the MRoE seem to have been contentious:

> initially we were told it was just for international healthcare workers – that didn't make sense.

Ultimately, the MRoE gave the medical commander discretion to admit local health care workers (capacity permitting) (Bricknell *et al.*, 2015).

Even taking into account that this ETU was only part of the UK response in Sierra Leone, the principles behind the MRoE and the resulting order of priority (international workers over local workers) seem controversial. According to a WHO report published in May 2015 (WHO, 2015) the local health service work-force had borne the brunt of the outbreak, being disproportionately affected (being 21–32 times more likely to be infected than the general population). In Sierra Leone, 368 of the country's health care workers were infected and 69 per cent of these died. Nurses and nurses' aides represented 57 per cent of this number and the country also lost some of its most significant medical leaders, such as virologist Dr Sheik Umar Khan. There was a real risk that the country's already-fragile health service would be completely decimated, hampering the country's recovery for years to come. It is therefore difficult to see why health care workers were not granted greater entitlement under the MRoE, notwith-standing the difficulties of determining how broadly 'health care worker' should be defined for this purpose.

The use of cameras in the ETU

One of the measures developed to minimize the risk to personnel in the ETU was a system of CCTV cameras (Bricknell *et al.*, 2015), with two-way commu-nications capability. According to our field work, the cameras had four broad potential uses:

- They enabled patients to be constantly monitored without the need for staff to be present at all times in areas where those suspected or confirmed to have EVD were being cared for (the so-called 'red zone').
- They enabled team leaders to determine how many staff of what kind to send into the red zone if a patient was in unexpected need of assistance. For example, it would enable the monitor to see whether a patient had hit his or her head when falling. This would reduce the number of staff needed to enter the red zone to attend to the patient.
- They enabled the monitoring of staff; team leaders could observe staff for e.g. signs of fatigue or potentially risky practice with a view to advising them to leave the red zone or offer advice on practice using two-way radios.
- They enabled infection control staff to potentially investigate the source of any infection to personnel by enabling them to 'follow' the actions of that member of staff in the period leading up to them becoming unwell with a view to improving infection control process.

The introduction of cameras was not however uncontroversial. Despite the advantages outlined above, there were concerns that their use violated the privacy of patients. These kinds of concern are not unfamiliar when surveillance technology is used in health care (see, for instance, Draper and Sorell (2013) and

Sorell and Draper (2012)). The view taken during design of operating procedures for the ETU was that the use of cameras within the ETU was no more than a more modern way of looking through a window at a patient, with the advantage of being able to converse with the patient using the two-way microphone system. The opportunity to interact from a distance when dealing with such a dangerous pathogen provided an additional layer of force protection to staff. In the event, patients were subsequently asked what they thought about the use of CCTV and feedback was that they felt reassured that they were being monitored and felt that if they needed assistance CCTV provided a robust adjunct to staff intervention.[3] Much ethical consideration was given both by the training team and by the deploying command team to the use of the video data that was captured as a component of the technical makeup of the CCTV system. Consideration had to be given to the collection of video imagery of patients (including some in great distress) and whether and when staff safety was outweighed by patient dignity. The decision-making process for this was handed over as a command decision to the command team within the ETU.

Whether or not concerns about patient privacy are justified rather depends on whether the capture of images was a proportionate response, how the resulting images are used and whether the data is stored. The conditions that pertained in the ETU were challenging. The working temperatures were exacerbated by the need for PPE, and it was not possible for staff to remain in the unit for more than a couple of hours before becoming exhausted, dehydrated and prone to errors that may have resulted in a breach of PPE or harm to their patients. These gruelling conditions, taken together with the legal obligation to minimize the risks to staff (see above), meant ETU policy and practice was designed to restrict entry into the red zone to that which was strictly necessary. 'Strictly necessary' was of course not a threshold intended to limit the treatment and care of patients who need it. 'Hands-on' care was provided when needed, but where 'hands-on' care was not required, just 'eyes-on' care, this 'eyes-on' care was provided at a distance using CCTV. This does not seem objectionable from the point of view of the provision of care. Some MSF units appear, from pictures at any rate, to have been designed so that patients could be monitored through Perspex screens on either side of a central corridor. One difference between the two systems was the amount of time it would take to get staff to a patient in need, since in the camera system PPE would need to be donned prior to entry. Keeping staff in PPE while not needed in the unit would have reduced entry time, but not the physical wear and tear of being encased in impervious garments. On the other hand, the camera system meant that someone had 'eyes on' the patient all of the time, whereas other systems depend on a member of staff to be present when a need arises, unless all patients are nursed in open Nightingale-style wards, which compromise privacy in different ways and increase the difficulties of infection control.

There is an obvious trade-off to be made between being monitored all of the time (CCTV) and having periods of privacy during which need may go unnoticed (having a greater staff presence in the red zone). One difference is that patients, assuming they were not too ill to notice, would know when there is someone nearby but would not know if, who and when someone is watching them on the camera. The use of CCTV increased the possibility of someone who might not otherwise have entered the red zone inadvertently violating privacy, for example someone not related to direct health care entering the office where the CCTV screens were. This inadvertent violation could however be readily limited by restricting access to the office.

In terms of proportionality, however, given that patients are generally subject to a degree of scrutiny even when direct care is not being provided, the additional intrusion on privacy is a small burden compared to the burdens and risks to the staff of the monitoring alternatives, particularly if these risks to staff would have knock-on effects on the care received by patients.

Whether it would be privacy-violating for the CCTV system to record as well as transmit images again probably depends on who accesses those images and for what purpose. Being able to revisit, for example, the moment a patient fell could be directly beneficial to the patient in terms of gaining a complete history. Revisiting CCTV images of an infected member of staff as part of an investigation of the source of their EVD infection would mean the member of staff and not the patients being observed, though it may be impossible not to see patients too (much like ordinary citizens might be viewed by police retracing the movement of a suspect through a crowd). Clearly, different people hold different views about the extent to which such surveillance activities are intrusive, and one clear difference is that a patient's bed-space is not a public area in the same way that e.g. a shopping mall or street is. However, in both cases the images are not being perused out of idle curiosity or some variety of prurient interest. Rather, there is a legitimate interest in play. Health care practitioners have an interest in infection risks to them being minimized by improved infection control practice; and their employers have a legitimate interest in being able to discharge their legal obligation to mitigate as far as possible the risks to employees going about their duties.

Clearly, policies should be in place that ensure that images are not stored for longer than necessary and are securely destroyed, and to ensure that access to stored images is limited to legitimate purposes. The consent of patients should be secured before stored images are used for training or other purposes.

Evacuation of EVD-infected personnel

Despite the WHO recommending that air travel should not be suspended, some groups lobbied hard to prevent all air travel from affected countries. There was debate, including in the UK, over repatriating affected nationals and the risk of transmission. Indeed, this seems to have been one of the rationale for establishing the DMS-run EVD treatment unit (Bricknell *et al.*, 2015). Accordingly, it was not clear – particularly in the run up to the initial deployment – whether military personnel who became infected could or would be brought back to the UK, including being repatriated for burial if they succumbed to the virus.

This raised two issues: first, whether there was a moral obligation to evacuate military personnel back to the UK for treatment (or burial); and, second, in face of the uncertainty over whether staff could or would be brought home, what information should be provided to deploying personnel on this issue.

Was there an obligation to undertake to evacuate infected military personnel?

During Operation HERRICK (the codename given to British operations in Afghanistan 2001–14), care provided to injured soldiers was improved by the establishment of a well-equipped Role Three hospital in Camp Bastion and also the increase in skills and techniques forged through experience of treating the wounded between 2006 and 2014 (Hodgetts, 2014). One aspect of this care was the rapid evacuation of the British wounded, by the Royal Air Force (RAF) Critical Care Air Support Team, for definitive care in the UK. Likewise, those who were killed in action were repatriated for burial with full military honours (Walklate *et al.*, 2015), which was not historically the case. The Commonwealth War Graves Commission maintains 23,000 cemeteries and memorials in 154 countries that commemorate soldiers who were buried where they fell in combat zones. The routine evacuation of the injured and dead of Operation HERRICK may have created a cultural *expectation* of repatriation but this expectation may not have a moral basis.

During the planning and first training stages for Operation GRITROCK, there was no policy for repatriation.

The Royal Free Hospital in London is the only high-level isolation unit in the UK and has only two beds. At the time that the planning for Operation GRITROCK was taking place, only one patient with EVD had been treated in the unit, a volunteer civilian nurse (Will Pooley) who had been repatriated by the RAF in August 2014. Accordingly, it was unclear whether there would be sufficient beds in the UK to evacuate infected military personnel to, or whether the standard of care provided in the UK would actually be superior to that planned in the EVD treatment unit (albeit that this care would be provided in more comfortable surroundings). Indeed, it might be contended that, given the experience of treating multiple EVD cases, the care provided in the unit would surpass that provided by the Royal Free. Moreover, as Bricknell *et al.* suggest,

> the goal for deploying the EVD TU [Ebola Virus Disease Treatment Unit] was to demonstrably deliver a level of care to infected healthcare workers … as close as practicable to that provided in Western national infectious disease containment facilities.
>
> (Bricknell *et al.*, 2015)

This suggests two things. The most obvious is an expectation that the standard of care would in fact be very good. But, second, confidence in that standard may conceivably have been undermined, rather than demonstrated, if those staffing the facility were routinely removed for care elsewhere. Moreover, there was the additional question of whether repatriation was the right thing to do given the potential risk of transmission to the UK, which would pose a risk of harm to the general civilian population.

Michael Gross (2008) has argued that military personnel who cannot be rehabilitated for battlefield duties fall outside the concern of military medicine and become the concern of civilian medical services, where they should not be regarded as a higher priority for treatment than civilians with similar health needs. This argument assumes that the military medical effort at the time is concentrated on sustaining the fighting force, which is an assumption that may not be appropriate in cases of *humanitarian* military intervention such as Operation GRITROCK. Nonetheless, Gross's argument appears, at least at first sight, to have some relevance in the circumstances of Operation GRITROCK. Here the military medics were deployed to the ETU, as part of a humanitarian effort, to treat – at least in the first instance – *civilian* health care workers. The 'enemy' was the virus and the 'troops' were the 'coalition' of health care workers, local and international, treating the affected local population. By analogy, then, those who should be prioritized for treatment in the ETU should have been those 'troops' most like to return to the 'front line' of treating EVD patients. Indeed, such 'troops' would be arguably more effective since they would have immunity from further infection. Given that the predicted British military tour of duty was between 60–90 days (depending on role), it seems unlikely that any British military personnel who recovered from EVD would realistically have continued to work in the unit. Local health care workers, on the other hand, could reasonably have been expected to return to work upon recovery. The situation in relation to the expatriate civilian volunteer workers is less clear: some may have chosen to return to work on the 'front line' (Will Pooley returned to Sierra Leone following his successful treatment). Others may have chosen repatriation (or simply come to the end of their agreed period of volunteering). This line of argument suggests that the correct order of priority for the British military medics in the ETU (see MRoE above) should have been first to treat the local health care workers, then any international workers likely to remain in Sierra Leone on recovery, with the British military and international workers unlikely to remain in country being third in line. If, on the other hand, the battle being fought was that of combatting the fear of international civilian responders (as the 'mission' reported by Bricknell *et al.* 2015 suggests) then the prioritization of international workers may have been justified, though infected British forces would have remained in third position (since they had no choice but to go if ordered to).

Gross (2008) also argues that not providing sophisticated treatment to wounded service personnel (who cannot be returned to battle) is unlikely to have negative impact on morale. He argues that '[a]bandonment is probably more corrosive of morale than lack of sophisticated care' because the 'cries of the wounded left on the battlefield were probably far more demoralising for an army than anything the enemy could throw at them' (Gross, 2008, p. 5). Bien, Kinoshita and Rosen (2008) respond to this point by suggesting that not being able to offer care to the 'unsalvagable' wounded may undermine the morale of the military *medics* (if not the troops generally). They contend that 'one core motivator for the United States military is their commitment to comrades' and that '[a]s members of the military, it is likely that blocking a helping professionals' ability to assist their comrades would result in burnout and compassion fatigue' (Bien *et al.*, 2008, p. 22). If they are correct, and if the same motivations can be applied to the British military, then expecting the medics in the ETU not to prioritize the care of their infected co-workers might be equally damaging.

Selgelid argues that when

> volunteers suffer injury in the pursuit of selfless activity, they deserve compensation from the societies they serve. A principle of reciprocity would hold that when volunteers make sacrifices for the sake of society, it is right to expect society to give them something back in return.
>
> (Selgelid, 2008, p. 19)

He continues that, while soldiers injured in the discharge of their duties are clearly owed what Gross (2008) categorizes as a right to health care on the grounds of their humanity – just like anyone else – they may have additional rights that are generated from reciprocity. To fail to recognize this by prioritizing them over citizens in equal need of care is to unfairly place all of burdens of the 'health harms' of war onto soldiers. The UK Armed Forces Covenant (MOD, 05/11) in part reflects Selgelid's position by stating that, in recognition of society's moral obligation to its armed forces, those *injured while on duty* should get priority care. It is a little more ambiguous, however, when it comes to veterans: 'veterans … should receive priority treatment where it relates to a condition that results from their service in the Armed Forces, subject to clinical need' (MOD, 05/11). Selgelid-type reciprocity arguments would, however, apply equally well to anyone who volunteers (even if as a paid worker) to care for those with EVD, so it may not help to determine priority within even a military-run ETU. It may, however, bring duties of reciprocity to bear when considering whether or not to repatriate military (or other) personnel for treatment when this runs the risk of transmission to the home nation.

Repatriation that runs the risk of transmission may equate to sharing the burdens of the health harms of the response to EVD with the home population, who would be otherwise sheltered from these harms. On the other hand, if one of the aims of deploying the military was to attempt to contain EVD in West Africa, rather than sharing the health harms of the fight against EVD, repatriation potentially brings the fight itself home. In this respect, then, what the volunteers (military or otherwise) might be sacrificing for the sake of others is not just the effort they expend abroad, or even just their health or their lives. They would also be taking on the *additional* burden of *not* being able to be repatriated for treatment. The magnitude of this burden depends upon the quality of the care being offered in the ETU (in our case, remember, the standard of care was assumed to be very good). Moreover, there may be a motivational difference between the military and civilian deployees. Military deployees are ordered to deploy and the motivation for deploying belongs to their government (which may or may not have primarily been the protection of the – in this case – British population by containing EVD in West Africa). We might suppose civilian volunteers to be primarily motivated by the plight of those in West Africa, in which case it is the EVD-affected population who might be regarded as having some kind of reciprocal duty. Returning to the military deployees, if repatriation is not possible then the reciprocal duty may need to be met in other ways, for instance through compensation or prioritization for ongoing care back home once repatriation without risk of transmission is possible.

As things turned out, only one of those deployed to the ETU was infected. The infected individual and five close contacts were repatriated in early March for treatment and observation respectively. In addition, at the end of January 2015 two serving health care workers sustained needle-stick injuries in the EVD TU and were also evacuated (Bricknell *et al.*, 2016).

Should the debate about repatriation be shared with those deploying?

So much for treatment and repatriation. Our second issue regarding the possible evacuation was whether this uncertainty over repatriation should have been shared during pre-deployment training. Our field observations and preparatory interviews suggest a reluctance to have a full and frank exchange with deployees in answer to their questions about evacuation. One reason for this was that, because there was uncertainty, those being questioned felt that they had no definite information to share and were understandably reluctant to give, or even appear to give, false reassurances. Another concern related to this was that sharing uncertainty may itself undermine morale, particularly in the less experienced junior ranks. This was also an issue in relation to discussing the risk of infection, which was also something of an unknown. This type of concern is another example of the tension that the dual obligations of a military career give health care workers. Certainly, the norms in health care practice point to a full and frank disclosure of information, including not shying away from the technically difficult communication of information about uncertainty and risk. Equally, maintaining the trust and confidence of troops is important in the military. There is arguably a case for maintaining a position of 'honest but less than full disclosure' where those receiving the information have little scope for autonomous decision-making, and loss of confidence may undermine operational effectiveness. Whether this line of reasoning is as justified in the face of non-combat risks may depend on how swayed one is by the arguments elsewhere in this collection that this kind of operation, because of its nature, should have been conducted on a volunteer-only basis. At the time, there was very little time to devote to peripheral issues such as this one during the planning phase for Operation GRITROCK. The training given to the first set of deploying troops was devised and delivered within a matter of weeks. It is, however, a topic that the military might like to reflect on as they begin to absorb the lessons of this deployment and plan for future operations.

Conclusion

Operation GRITROCK was the first purely humanitarian mission that the UK military had undertaken for some years, and, as a consequence, planning for this deployment raised some new ethical challenges. These ranged from bigger picture questions about what the role and the purpose of the mission was, to specific issues like how to the balance the privacy of patients against the safety of medical personnel. This project has helped to identify and explore issues to facilitate the creation of training materials to help those deploying on similar missions in the future, so that they can benefit from the experiences of those on Operation GRITROCK. A partial, illustrative example of this ongoing work has been included in this chapter. If anyone reading this chapter would like to contribute to this ongoing work they are invited to make contact with the first author or the editors of this collection.

Example of case-based training materials generated from the reported experience

The process

One of the aims of our project was to create training materials to prepare military personnel for the ethical challenges they might face, initially on Operation GRITROCK but also more broadly when deployed on humanitarian missions. For the most part, we are working on developing case studies for discussion based on the experiences of those who worked in the Kerry Town ETU. We have used the experiences of participants to create these, but have generated composite cases to preserve anonymity.

Working on the assumption that those involved in medical military policy, planning and governance might benefit from some exposure to ethical issues, we included the issues discussed here in our expanding portfolio.

The cases will, as far as possible, be publicly available. We have therefore also been working with members of the COST action 'Disaster Bioethics' on these cases, and we have also piloted them at the 2015 DMS Ethics Symposium. The format is a brief case study with questions for group discussion.

A sample:

The case: cameras replacing carers?

A treatment unit is being set up as part of a humanitarian effort to combat an outbreak of a severe and infectious virus in a low-income country. The affected country is hot and humid. Staff are only able to work for a couple of hours in personal protective equipment (PPE) owing to the extreme heat and humidity as there is no possibility of effective air conditioning. It is possible for cameras to be fixed in the treatment areas of those affected by, or suspected of having, the virus. This would enable staff to monitor patients without having to don PPE and be exposed to risk by entering the 'red zone' (the area where there is risk of infection). Fixing cameras would enable patients to be monitored remotely.

The feed from the cameras could be recorded. This would enable staff to decide how many personnel to send in to a patient needing care (e.g. if the patient collapses and falls, it would be possible to replay the tape to see whether they hit their head or if a patient is agitated). A potential longer-term use for the recordings would be retracing the movements of anyone working in the unit who succumbs to infection. This could potentially improve infection control routines and also assist training back in the sponsoring nation's training facility. The recording of patients could, however, be regarded as an intrusion of privacy and a failure to respect dignity. The use of recorded data for purposes other than patient care might also be regarded as a misuse of personal data.

Please discuss the following questions with your group members:

1   Using an ethical framework that focuses on consequences, list and discuss the arguments for and against using camera in this way.
2   Taking the perspective that 'our duties to our patient come first' list and discuss arguments for and against using cameras in this way.
3   Compare the arguments that you have generated. Note whether and if so why some arguments appear in both exercises. Which set of arguments do you find most persuasive and why?
4   What is your overall view about this use of cameras? Do you think your views have changed during the course of this exercise? Reflect on what changed your views.
5   If using cameras is an acceptable response, should there be any limits to the use of cameras? If so, what and where? Who should be able to view the recordings?
6   Should patients' consent be gained? At what point? Should the patients be allowed to refuse consent and still receive treatment in the unit?
7   What should happen, and why, if a patient is admitted to the unit who is unable to give consent (lacks capacity)?
8   To what extent would you be prepared to impinge upon an individual's liberty and privacy by overruling their autonomy for 'the greater good'?
9   Is consent required from the staff too as all of their movements will also be recorded?

Issues raised by the case

1   Patients' right to privacy and dignity
2   Justifiable breaches to patients' privacy
3   Minimizing risk to staff by compromising individual patient care

Potential learning outcomes

1 Identification and consideration of ethical issues
2 Increased understanding of ethical issues and duties
3 Beginning to understand and apply consequentialist ways of addressing issues and associated problems
4 Beginning to understand how ethical issues may be anticipated and avoided

Sample of Tutor Guidance Notes:

Question 1

Using an ethical framework that focuses on consequences, examine the arguments for and against using cameras.

Arguments FOR:

Monitoring patients and their needs without having to go into the unit:

1 lessens the risk of infection to staff as staff are able to assess what is needed without having to enter the 'red zone' to determine patient needs;
2 reduces staff discomfort and the need to work in PPE in extreme heat and humidity where/when not necessary;
3 means less time in PPE, which might equate to less staff fatigue/stress and risk of associated mistakes in clinical care and infection control;
4 means that there is increased monitoring of patients. Any patient's needs should be easily observable and therefore clinical care can be more responsive and therefore improved;
5 means that there is a record of infection control measures taken. This may prove a useful tool in tracking possible routes of infection/risk of infection;
6 means that there is a record of treatment of patients with EVD. Can be used for future training and research purposes.

Arguments AGAINST:

Monitoring patients and their needs by cameras:

1 treats patients as objects of surveillance rather than people, which may translate directly into how staff then treat patients;
2 means that staff may spend less time with patients and patients will consequently feel uncared for;
3 might make staff nervous and they may make more mistakes and therefore increase their risk of infection and infection spread;
4 may be perceived by the local population and further populations as intrusive and undesirable and it may lead to a loss of trust in health care workers/ military in the UK;

> 5   may make patients feel that their rights have not been respected as they
>   haven't been asked about the cameras. Staff may also perceive either that the
>   ethical norm of the doctrine of informed consent has not been complied with,
>   or that if patients' consent has been sought it is conditional in that no treat-
>   ment is available without the use of cameras. This may be perceived as coer-
>   cive and 'big brotherish' and counter to the concept of patient autonomy. This
>   may also erode trust and confidence in the service being provided.

Acknowledgement

This work was supported by the Economic and Social Research Council (grant number ES/M011763/1) and the Royal Centre for Defence Medicine (Academia and Research).

Notes

1 A concise account of the support given by the Defence Medical Services to Operation GRITROCK has been published by Bricknell *et al.* (2015).
2 The Canadian military, for instance, has organisational responsibility for Canadian Disaster Assistance Response Team (DART), whose scope includes the provision of primary health care services. See www.forces.gc.ca/en/operations-abroad-recurring/dart.page.
3 Informal patient interviews conducted by Commander 2nd Medical Brigade, Brigadier K Beaton in November 2014 (personal correspondence).

References

Bien, G. D., Kinoshita, L. M. and Rossen, A. C. 2008. Need versus salvage; a health professional's perspective. *American Journal of Bioethics*, 8(2), 21–23.

Bricknell, M., Terrell, A., Ross, D. and White, D. 2016. Health protection during the Ebola crisis: the Defence Medical Services approach. *Journal of the Royal Army Medical Corps*, doi:10.1136/jramc-2015–000516.

Bricknell, M., Hodgetts, T., Beaton, K. and McCourt, A. 2015. Operation GRITROCK: the Defence Medical Services story and the emerging lessons from supporting the UK response to the Ebola Crisis. *Journal of the Royal Army Medical Corps*, doi: 10.1136/jramc-2015–000512.

Butler, D. 2014. Models overestimate Ebola cases. *Nature*, 515(18), doi:10.1038/515018a.

Connor, P., Bailey, M., Tuck, J. J., Green, A. and Hodgetts, T. 2015. UK Defence Medical Services Ebola Treatment Facility. *The Lancet*, 385(9969), 685–686.

Curtin, P. 1990. The end of 'the white man's grave': Nineteenth century mortality in west Africa. *The Journal of Interdisciplinary History*, 21(31), 63–88.

Draper, H. and Sorell, T. 2013. Telecare, remote monitoring and care. *Bioethics*, 27(7), 365–372.

Gov.uk. 2014. *How the UK Government Is Responding to Ebola*. Available online at www.gov.uk/government/topical-events/ebola-virus-government-response/about (accessed 27 November 2016).

Gross, M. L. 2008. Why treat the wounded? Warrior care, military salvage and national health. *American Journal of Bioethics*, 8(2), 3–12.

Her Majesty's Government. 2015. *National Security Strategy and Strategic Defence and Security Review 2015*. London: HMSO. Available online at www.gov.uk/government/uploads/system/uploads/attachment_data/file/555607/2015_Strategic_Defence_and_Security_Review.pdf (accessed 27 November 2016).

Hodgetts, T. J. 2014. A roadmap for innovation. *Journal of the Royal Army Medical Corps*, doi:10.1136/jramc-2014-000250.

Little, A. 2010. The brigadier who saved Sierra Leone. Available online at http://news.bbc.co.uk/1/hi/programmes/from_our_own_correspondent/8682505.stm (accessed 8 January 2016).

Médecins Sans Frontières. 2014, 2 September. *Global Bio-disasters Response Urgently Needed in Ebola Fight*. Press Release. Available online at www.doctorswithoutborders.org/news-stories/press-release/global-bio-disaster-response-urgently-needed-ebola-fight (accessed 27 November 2016).

Ministry of Defence. 05/11. *The Armed Forces Covenant*. London: HMSO. Available online at www.gov.uk/government/uploads/system/uploads/attachment_data/file/49469/the_armed_forces_covenant.pdf (accessed 17 January 2016).

Office for the Coordination of Humanitarian Affairs. 2007. *Guidelines on the Use of Foreign Military and Civil Defence Assets in Disaster Relief*. Available online at www.unocha.org/what-we-do/coordination-tools/UN-CMCoord/publications (accessed 17 January 2016).

Renton, A. 2010. Sierra Leone: one place where Tony Blair remains an unquestioned hero. *Observer*, 18 April. Available online at www.theguardian.com/world/2010/apr/18/sierra-leone-international-aid-blair (accessed 8 January 2016).

Richards, D. 2014. *Taking Command*. London: Headline.

Selgelid, M. J. 2008. Just liability and reciprocity reasons for treating wounded soldiers. *American Journal of Bioethics*, 8(2), 19–20.

Sorell, T. and Draper, H. 2012. Telecare, surveillance and the welfare state. *American Journal of Bioethics*, 12(9), 36–44.

UNAIDS. Available online at www.unaids.org/en/regionscountries/countries/sierraleone.

UNICEF. Available online at www.unicef.org/infobycountry/sierraleone_statistics.html.

Walklate, S., Mythen, G. and McGarry, R. 2015. 'When you see the lipstick kisses …' – military repatriation, public mourning and the politics of respect. *Palgrave Communications*, 1, 15009.

World Health Organization. 2015. *Health Care Worker Infections in Guinea, Liberia and Sierra Leone: A Preliminary Report*. Available online at www.who.int/hrh/documents/21may2015_web_final.pdf (accessed 8 November 2015).

2 The Ebola response team deployment in the Republic of Guinea

Organizational, ethical, legal issues and a problem of responsibility

Ivan Kholikov and Kira Sazonova

Introduction

In accordance with the decision of the President of the Russian Federation, the Ministry of Defence of the Russian Federation was tasked to deploy to the Republic of Guinea in order to establish a military field hospital for infectious diseases. The hospital was sponsored by the Russian Federation to assist the Republic of Guinea in its fight against the Ebola epidemic. The hospital was originally designed to treat 200 patients suffering from infections such as cholera, plague, typhoid and Ebola and Marburg virus diseases. The hospital only contained 100 beds in order to ensure the proper sanitary epidemiological regime to avoid the spread of infection.

This chapter focuses on the results of the activity of the Russian Ebola response team in the Republic of Guinea, which posed many organizational, ethical and legal challenges. Particular attention is paid to the international legal issues that arise from pandemic diseases. Chief among these is the difficulty of assigning responsibility in an international environment where numerous actors are involved as well as agreeing on a mechanism to decide the relevant international institutional jurisdictions that are authorized to establish liability.

Organizational issues

The Surgeon General of the Russian Federation Armed Forces was ordered to deploy a group of specialists to form the Ebola response team with the aim of establishing a hospital and training local health care workers to operate it. The main tasks of the Russian mission were to admit into the hospital patients suspected of having Ebola, diagnose cases of Ebola, organize treatment of infected patients and conduct anti-epidemic measures to prevent the further spread of infection.

The mission encountered a number of challenges with the most acute being numerous and varied organizational issues. Upon the arrival of the Russian mission by plane it became clear that nobody was expecting the mission despite prior diplomatic correspondence and agreements. There was nobody ready to unload the planes, refuel them or carry out other necessary administrative procedures. After a period of time, a representative from the Russian Aluminium Company (RusAL) helped by providing the necessary people to arrange the required personnel for unloading the planes and safeguarding the equipment. The Russian Embassy also assisted by contacting the local health care authorities that enabled the mission to complete all the required legal procedures for handing over the large and expensive equipment.

After the arrival of the Minister of Health, who signed all the required formal documents, the hospital was stockpiled at the RusAL depots located in the vicinity of Conakry. The materials remained there owing to the high level of risk that the hospital would have been robbed, which regularly occurs with humanitarian aid that arrives into the country without proper controls for stockpiling and further distribution. This problem is widespread and the high volumes of aid arriving in Guinea has led to a black market in the selling and reselling of humanitarian aid. This is exacerbated by corruption among authorities, which has resulted in very few resources reaching the people.

The march to Kindia, the planned location for the hospital, took almost 20 hours owing to the very poor road conditions and the necessity to provide proper security measures. Again, there was very little assistance from the local side and RusAL organized almost everything. To avoid complications at all levels, especially when dealing with the local population, the Russian mission stressed that it was there to assist the people of the Republic of Guinea to fight epidemics of various diseases, including some hemorrhagic fevers endemic in the area. This approach appeared to be sensible because, once the mission had arrived and began to work, many local people approached to ask whether the purpose of the mission was to deal with Ebola or not. The most important factor that contributed to the overall security of the hospital was its proximity to the military unit of the Guinean army. The Minister of Health, who was himself a Colonel and a former Surgeon General of the Guinea Army, personally contributed a lot to that. The hospital was officially set up and handed over to the Guinean authorities on 19 December 2014. Following the official handover there was a visit by ministers from the Republic of Guinea, where all the equipment and facilities were demonstrated.

The World Health Organization (WHO) had been operational in Guinea since the beginning of the Ebola outbreak. Despite the good work carried out by the WHO, the Russian mission sometimes had the impression that it also contributed a lot to the paranoia that surrounded the problem. Ebola had been present in the region for many years and was never previously considered an issue that posed a threat to international security and stability although the spread of the disease beyond West Africa was a cause for concern. It seemed that once again there was a media panic on the likelihood of a full-blown Ebola pandemic similar to the recent outbreaks of SARS and especially H1N1 and H5N1 influenzas.

Ethical challenges

Rather than ethical challenges connected with Ebola in particular, the Russian mission was most disturbed by the desperate levels of poverty and unemployment and the anti-sanitary environment. The absence of a functioning sewage system in the capital of the country meant that the waste from two million people simply floated out into the ocean, where children enjoyed swimming and washing themselves. Instead of pavements, the streets were covered with pressed garbage. In such an environment, it is not surprising that you come across diseases that are not so prevalent elsewhere in the world today such as cholera, typhoid and many others. However, these more entrenched problems were never the central focus of the WHO.

An important piece of advice offered by the Russian ambassador was to avoid mentioning the word 'Ebola'. The ambassador recalled an incident involving the US and British missions, who wanted to set up a hospital for Ebola patients in Conakry. There was a big event planned, with ambassadors invited to lay the cornerstone of the hospital, when an angry crowd armed with stones and sticks appeared and destroyed everything. It appeared that the local people were sure that Ebola did not exist and they were confident that people from the West brought this disease to their country to exterminate them in order to obtain access to their natural resources. This went some way to explain the frequent unwillingness of the local community to cooperate in such situations when their cooperation was indispensable. Having access to the high-level political figures made it possible to overcome some barriers on the lower levels; nevertheless, it took a considerable amount of time for the local authorities to take a decision on where to set up the hospital. It was a place near a town of Kindia, 150 km from the capital in the direction of the Guinean forest, which is considered Ebola's natural breeding ground.

The lectures conducted by representatives of the Russian mission on how to operate the hospital, on the approaches towards dealing with outbreaks of extremely dangerous infections and on other topics were well attended by many highly educated medical professionals who asked good questions and showed an interest and a dedication to fight the outbreak. But, when Russian specialists asked the Minister of Health to send three specialists to be shown how to work on site, nobody came. The ethical issue of treating patients with experimental drugs is also extremely difficult, but the mission concluded that in situations where the alternative for a patient is death it can be ethically appropriate.

Another ethical challenge was the huge amount of false information surrounding the problem of Ebola in general. The available information, mainly obtained from the Internet and mass media, gave the strong impression that it was unlikely that the members of the mission would leave without having contracted Ebola. Upon arrival, the mission discovered that there were no dead bodies lining the roads, as is the case in horror films, and that the inhabitants of city went about their normal daily life, both during the day and at night. There were some warning banners in the streets and in the airport with precautions advised in certain places, mainly encouraging individuals to measure their temperature as well as undertake simple hygiene measures such as washing hands. The tropic temperatures of more than 35{degree}C meant that wearing anti-plague suits or any other kind of protection would have looked out of place, while ignoring shaking hands with other people would have caused them to turn away from us. The mission realized that the best approach was to ignore their concerns and to live as normal a life as possible while paying special attention to hygiene measures. While working in Guinea the mission received phone calls from the press service of the Russian Ministry of Defence, asking, 'Are you surviving? How is the epidemic? Are there really dying people lying under every tree?' This perfectly illustrated the misconception of the media outside the country with the reality on the ground.

Another issue, which is both ethical and legal, arises around the problem of quarantine, particularly as the incubation period for Ebola lasts 21 days. After returning from the Republic of Guinea, the mission was obliged to spend only nine days under observation in accordance with the recommendation of Chief Preventive Medicine Specialist of the Ministry of Defence. This did not amount to a classic quarantine with strict isolation, although strong restrictions were placed on the activities that the members of the mission were permitted to undertake. The RusAL personnel were obliged to spend all 21 days in quarantine, which was organized for the company in Morocco. The most important indication of the onset of Ebola is temperature, so the regular measurement of it was the only required medical procedure. One ethical issue that did arise in this respect was the exposure of others during transit. Rather than taking a military flight out of the country, the mission flew back on regular Air France flights via Paris to Moscow, upon which all passengers had to fill out special forms designed by WHO and hand them over to the crew for further processing by health care workers. Since the final destination of the mission was Saint Petersburg, they had to take a connection in Moscow, where they were interviewed before proceeding further. After landing in Saint Petersburg, the plane was moved to a remote parking lot, where employees from the State Preventive Medicine Service (a civilian body) entered the plane and started distributing the WHO forms. When passengers, especially in business class, started protesting against the waste of their time in filling in unnecessary forms, they were told that nobody would leave the plane before all forms were collected because there were some passengers on board who had come from West Africa. This possible exposure of other passengers to the disease is an uncomfortable ethical issue and difficult to address in circumstances where public travel is necessary.

Before moving to the legal challenges, it is worth mentioning that Ebola remains a real challenge, and that we must pay tribute to those people who were and still are assisting those who suffer from this very real threat. The issues of pandemics and mass diseases are widely discussed in political contest, being considered a part of various conspiracy theories that tend to see them as a source of reaching some specific political goals.

Legal issues

Diseases and epidemics: legal dimension

As various pandemics, including haemorrhagic fevers such as Ebola, often (if not always) transcend national jurisdiction and affect many countries, questions of responsibility are very acute. These can centre upon which actor – the state or international organizations – has responsibility for actions or non-actions to avoid the global spread of such diseases. We would like to examine the problems posed by epidemics and mass diseases and consider these issues from the perspective of international law. The most important factor for referring the particular outbreak to the international legal sphere is the sufficient criteria for giving official status to a particular threat.

The exact figures may vary significantly, but, based on the practice of the last 15 years, it is possible to state that both the UN and the WHO started to talk about any pandemic as a threat to international security when the number of people affected exceeded 2,000 across five or more states. As far as particular diseases are concerned, the International Health Regulations define a disease as an 'illness or medical condition, irrespective of origin or source, that presents or could present significant harm to humans' (World Health Organization 2005, p. 7). Such diseases include cholera, plague, haemorrhagic fevers and some other significant infectious diseases that are endemic in certain regions.

The most active attempts to elaborate a unified legal approach to this problem were taken almost at the same time as the UN International Law Commission completed the Draft Articles on the Responsibility of States for Internationally Wrongful Acts. The SARS outbreak in South East Asia in 2003 was the first case to lead to concern over the problems that mass diseases posed as threats to international and regional security. According to the WHO, the number of people suffering from SARS exceeded 3,000 and the disease affected 24 states (World Health Organization, 2003a).

International responsibility for the proliferation of epidemics and mass diseases: theoretical aspect

The process of forming the branch of international responsibility took a long time and extremely difficult, as for any process that involves fundamental legal categories and influences the legal paradigm of the whole international community.

The responsibilities of states usually cause many more significant problems in comparison with the responsibility of the individuals. After the conclusion of the Nuremberg trials, the French member of the Tribunal, Donnedieu de Vabres, stated that the Nuremberg sentence did not exclude the criminal responsibility of a state as a legal entity (Vabres 1947, p. 822). And that is a moot point, because, in the case of individual responsibility, the list of possible variants of punishment is much more varied than in the case of state responsibility. How is it possible to punish a state or to apply force to a state as a sovereign entity and as an abstract legal category?

A significant factor in the difficulty of holding states to account is the absence at the supranational level of an enforcement competence in contemporary international relations. An undoubtedly positive step in this sense was the fixing of preemptory norms in the UN Charter that would allow for the use of force. This epitomizes the major difference between classic international law, which is composed of dispositive norms, and contemporary international law based on imperative norms contained within the Charter.

In 1955, Garcia Amador, the first International Law Commission (ILC) special rapporteur on state responsibility, noted that 'it would be difficult to find a topic beset with greater confusion and uncertainty' (Amador 1957, p. 175). In fact, that can be said not only about state responsibility but international responsibility as a legal branch itself. Nowadays the situation remains essentially the same and, even though much has been done, much more remains to be done both in the theoretical and especially in the practical sense.

There are several reasons explaining and defining the present situation in the sphere of international responsibility, including international responsibility for the proliferation of epidemics and mass diseases. The first factor is the fact that during the last 100 years the international community has been resolving a set of painful questions, which significantly influence the process of the development of international responsibility. How is it possible to separate where the sovereignty of one state ends and the sovereignty of another state begins? Who can judge a state that seriously breached the norms of international law? And how is it possible to punish such a state? The ambiguity and complexity of the answers to these questions have led to complete confusion in the sphere of international responsibility. That is probably why this branch is developing slower than the other branches of international law. It is precisely the development of international responsibility that may present a way of neutralizing many destructive tendencies in international relations.

The second reason explaining the present situation in the sphere of state responsibility is the widespread politicization of issues connected with international responsibility. Unfortunately, the international community today is unable to resolve many questions at the global level simply by deferring the competency for such issues to supranational structures when national interests remain that hinder progress. All these factors explain why the branch of international responsibility has a fairly short history in comparison with other branches of international law, for example international maritime law or diplomatic law, which have been in a process of development for hundreds of years.

On 7 December 1953, the UN General Assembly adopted Resolution 799, which requested that the ILC start the codification of the principles of state responsibility. However, the reports of the first ILC special rapporteur, Garcia Amador, on this problem were only concerned with the question of responsibility for injuries to the persons or property of aliens (Amador 1957). As Professor Tunkin, one of the ILC members, said in 1959, in 'the third and fourth decades of the twentieth century, the question of State responsibility had been discussed from one point of view only' (United Nations 1959, 149).

Nevertheless, in the second half of the twentieth century some new institutions dealing with international responsibility began to develop – notably with respect to liability for damage caused by space objects and the liability for environmental violations. Moreover, there were also some attempts to analyse the problem of responsibility from the position of a particular region. Thus, in 1961 the Inter-American Juridical Committee adopted the *Contribution of the American Continent to the Principles of International Law that Govern the Responsibility of the State* report. As Roberto Ago wrote in 1969, 'The Committee also decided to confine its study to the practice of the Latin American countries, because in its opinion, only those countries had made a "contribution to the development of international law on the subject"' (Ago 1969, p. 129). However, the report did not produce particular resonance in the academic community.

In 1962, the ILC decided to continue uniting the different positions on the issue of state responsibility. The Italian Professor Ago was appointed special rapporteur, which began what is now called the 'Ago Revolution' (Pellet 2010, p. 11). Ago presented eight reports, which formed the foundation of the contemporary doctrine of international responsibility. He was preceded in the post in 1979 by Riphagen and Arangio-Ruiz, who were appointed in 1979 and 1988, respectively, and also produced a number of reports. It wasn't until Crawford was appointed special rapporteur in 1996 that a compromise was found, and in 2001 the Draft Articles on Responsibility of States for Internationally Wrongful Acts was adopted. However, Crawford understood that the result was that the draft became 'rigorously general in character' (Crawford 2002, p. 2). Despite the generality of the articles, it can be argued that such a result was better than nothing and, even though they were only recommendations, rather than legally binding, they represented a significant step on the way to building and strengthening the law of responsibility. Indeed all of the reports of the special rapporteurs contributed to the conceptualization and development of international responsibility and exhibited different doctrinal approaches to this topic.

Besides the reports of the special rapporteurs, in the reporting period the problem of international responsibility was intensively discussed in the works of Carella (1985), Caron (1998), Dupuy (1990), Greafrath (1993) and Vitta (1953). They also provided strong theoretical support for the branch of international responsibility. Pellet went so far as to claim that: 'Responsibility is the corollary of international law, the best proof of its existence and the most credible measure of its effectiveness' (Pellet 2010, p. 3). Politicians and diplomats often laud international responsibility; however, when it comes to the practical realities of international relations such rhetoric is often rendered redundant. What is the situation we are faced with today? In fact, the branch of international responsibility has three main institutions: the responsibility of states, the responsibility of international organizations and individual responsibility. The latter is the most developed and codified compared to the others and is tightly intertwined with international criminal law: 'It is largely, if not exclusively, criminal' (Pellet 2010, p. 8).

After sharp debates in 2006, the ILC adopted the Draft Articles on the Responsibility of International Organizations. These now serve as a basis for the current guidelines relating to state responsibility as well as for the responsibility of international organizations. The result is logical – contemporary international relations are not strongly influenced by the necessity to observe obligations out of respect for responsibility or out of fear of responsibility. That is why international responsibility remains merely a draft, not a reality. Dupuy called the existing law of state responsibility 'the hostile jungle' (1999, p. 385), and so it is, with this also an apt term to characterize every legal institute dealing with international responsibility.

Apparently, it is not yet time to fully develop this branch of international law, because the international community is still not ready for it. We totally agree with Reuter that 'responsibility is at the heart of international law ... it constitutes an essential part of what may be considered the Constitution of the international community' (1995, p. 574). The development and codification of international responsibility can be coupled to the beginning of the Era of Sovereignty in 1648. Hopefully we have a chance to live in the Era of Responsibility.

International responsibility for the proliferation of epidemics and mass diseases: practical aspect

The important legal aspect is the consideration of actions or non-actions of certain states as the possible basis for international responsibility. The Draft Articles on Responsibility of States for Internationally Wrongful Acts are quite general in nature and contain only secondary legal norms. Nevertheless, analyses of their content can result in the conclusion that there is a connection between the actions of some states during pandemics with so-called *erga omnes* obligations. These are international obligations that the state voluntary undertakes within the world community. The UN International Criminal Court used this term for the first time in a resonance case, *Barcelona Traction* (Belgium against Spain), in 1970.

The topic of non-proliferation of epidemics and mass diseases is also closely connected with the term 'international public order'. Judge Manfred Lachs is considered to have coined the term, which is being actively worked out by the American school of international law (Criddle *et al.* 2008, p. 344). The idea of international public order is the cornerstone of the approach that 'the interests of the world community dominate over sovereignty wills and selfish interests of particular states' (Hsiung 2004, p. 16). However, as far as particular forms of realization of international responsibility in a case of a violation of *erga omnes* obligations by the state are concerned, the UN International Law Commission pointed out that this matter is too complicated to make a universal rule regarding compensation and therefore limited itself to drafting only the general principle.

A very important argument in favour of considering the non-proliferation of epidemics as *erga omnes* obligations of states is the content of the key international legal documents. For example, in accordance with Article 12 of the

International Covenant on Economic, Social and Cultural Rights of 1966, the states take obligations to ensure the health of their citizens by all necessary measures, which will allow them to conduct actions aimed at the 'prevention, treatment and control of epidemics, occupational and other diseases' (United Nations 1966, Paragraph 12).

In accordance with a commentary made by the UN Committee on Economic, Social and Cultural Rights,

> the states carry individual and collective responsibility for interaction in case of disasters and for provision of humanitarian aid in case of emergencies.... Taking into account that some diseases can easily overcome the state boarders, the international community bears collective responsibility in this situation.

The committee stressed in particular that 'economically developed States have special responsibility and interest to assist the poorer the developing States in this regard' (Office of the High Commissioner for Human Rights 2000, Paragraph 40).

It is evident that the perspective of holding the state to account for the spread of epidemics by addressing some international legal body, for example the UN International Court of Justice, is highly unlikely. A better option to establish international responsibility could be a joint commission where all interested states are represented.

The most problematic issue here is the determination of particular forms of international responsibility. According to the Draft Articles on Responsibility of States for Internationally Wrongful Acts, it is possible to identify three forms of such state responsibility: compensation, restitution and satisfaction.

But, owing to the fact that responsibility for actions or non-actions that led to the spread of a mass disease beyond its national borders is not only on the guilty party but also the victim, the realization of responsibility in such instances become much more complicated. The territory affected by the epidemic turns into a so-called 'estranging zone', owing to the considerable constraints imposed upon the movement of people and goods, which influences states' attractiveness for inward investment and as tourist destinations. For instance, in 2003 the WHO paid great attention to the various trading limitations imposed upon SARS-affected areas (World Health Organization, 2003b).

One more important issue on this subject is the question of whether there is an obligation of states to cooperate in the case of an epidemic, or whether states should be permitted to deal with these problems separately. The tendency over the last few years shows that the international community actively reacts in the case of pandemics, for example when the UN Security Council unanimously adopted Resolution 2177(2014) at an emergency meeting on the Ebola outbreak in West Africa. This resolution in its preamble declared the present outbreak a 'threat to international peace and security'. Furthermore, it called on countries to 'lift general travel and border restrictions' and 'provide urgent resources and assistance'. At the meeting, the secretary-general announced that the UN was to deploy an international emergency health mission called 'UN Mission for Ebola Emergency Response' (UNMEER, the first ever UN emergency health mission) with aims to stop the outbreak, treat the infected, ensure essential services, preserve stability and prevent further outbreaks in other states (UN News Center 2014a). He added that its effectiveness depended on the support of the international community.

On 19 September 2014, the UN General Assembly underlined its commitment to respond to the outbreak 'in a timely, effective and coordinated manner' in Resolution GA/11552. The Mexican representative considered the adoption to be 'a clear testimony of international cooperation'. On 22 September 2014, the UN set up the Ebola Response Multi-Partner Trust Fund, seeking contributions not only from member states but also from businesses and individuals. It also launched a website on the UN system's global response to the Ebola outbreak.

At the 'High-level Meeting on Response to the Ebola Virus Disease Outbreak' on 25 September 2014, Ban Ki-moon noted the 'overwhelming international political momentum for the UN to play a leading role in coordinating the global response' (UN News Center 2014b).

The responsibility of international organizations for the proliferation of epidemics and mass diseases

The problem of responsibility becomes more complicated when it comes to the responsibility of international organizations. For instance, in 2013 there was a major scandal connected with the epidemic of cholera in Haiti.

In October 2010, only a few months after the country had been devastated by a massive earthquake, Haiti was afflicted with another tragedy: the outbreak of a cholera epidemic that killed over 8,000 people and made more than 600,000 sick. Tragically, the cholera outbreak – the first in the modern Haitian history – was possibly caused by the United Nations peacekeeping troops, who inadvertently carried the disease from Nepal to the Haitian town of Maye. In October 2010, the UN deployed peacekeeping troops from Nepal to join the Mission for the Stabilization in Haiti (MINUSTAH). The UN stationed these troops at an outpost near Méyè, approximately 40 kilometres north-east of Haiti's capital, Port-au-Prince. The Méyè base was just a few metres from a tributary of the Artibonite River, the largest river in Haiti and one the country's main sources of water for drinking, cooking and bathing. Peacekeepers from Nepal, where cholera is endemic, arrived in Haiti shortly after a major outbreak.

There was a report compiled entitled *Peacekeeping without Accountability*, which provided a comprehensive analysis of the evidence that the UN troops brought cholera to Haiti, relevant international legal and humanitarian standards necessary to understand the UN accountability, and steps that the UN and other key national and international actors must take to rectify this harm (Transnational Development Clinic *et al.*, 2013).

Despite overwhelming evidence linking the MINUSTAH to the outbreak, the UN has denied responsibility for causing the epidemic. The organization has refused to adjudicate legal claims from cholera victims or to otherwise remedy the harms they have caused. By causing the epidemic and then refusing to provide redress to those affected, the UN has breached its commitments to the government of Haiti, its obligations under international law, and principles of humanitarian relief. Now, more than four years after the epidemic began, the UN is leading efforts to eliminate cholera but has still not taken responsibility for the actions of its peacekeepers. As new infections continue to mount, accountability for the UN's failures in Haiti is as important as ever.

Outrage over the negligence of the UN officials and peacekeepers, which is the most likely source of the cholera epidemic, which inflicted massive suffering and thousands of deaths in Haiti, is justified. However, there is another side of the coin: a successful lawsuit requiring the UN to pay compensation would not punish those directly responsible. Worse, it would likely lead to a reduction in UN field activities, which could lead to even broader suffering. Although the UN has a mixed record in peacekeeping and has played a role in several terrible tragedies, including Haiti, the world community has an interest in preserving the ability of the UN to respond to crises where particular nations are unwilling or unable to respond directly. Members of the UN Security Council also have a responsibility to try to prevent future tragedies and provide a remedy to those suffering from cholera in Haiti today. They can do this by advancing key reforms to UN procedures, enhancing the accountability of the UN and troop-contributing countries, leading an effort to reprogramme existing UN resources to assist anti-cholera efforts in Haiti, and using their privileged positions in the UN Security Council to more thoroughly scrutinize and vet UN operations.

Although the UN has almost certainly contributed to the terrible situation in Haiti, there are opinions that weakening the privileges and immunities of the UN in situations like Haiti should be opposed. The UN and its affiliated organizations are engaged in a multitude of activities that could result in casualties, property damage or other negative consequences. The Haiti lawsuit would set a precedent that could open up the organization to other claims that could impose an immense financial burden on the member states that pay the expenses of the organization (Schaefer, 2013).

As an illustration, if the UN agreed to pay full compensation and restitution to Haitians harmed by cholera, that is, paying the full $50,000 in claims allowed under Resolution 52/247 to the nearly 700,000 alleged victims in Haiti, payments would total more than $32 billion. This figure does not include possible claims arising from the spread of cholera from Haiti to other countries. Moreover, claims could possibly be much higher if the $50,000 limitation is not applicable. Resolution 52/247 endorses the view expressed in a 1997 Report of the Secretary-General that 'no financial limitations are proposed with regard to claims arising as a result of gross negligence or willful misconduct' (Knox, 2013).

Considering Haiti's low per capita income, many individual claims would certainly fall short of $50,000, and the extent of the damage in Haiti is extreme, but it does provide a stark demonstration of the potential financial exposure that allowing the lawsuit to proceed would create for an organization with 15 peacekeeping operations and numerous political missions and humanitarian projects around the world.

The potential impact of a successful legal case on future UN peacekeeping and humanitarian missions goes beyond financial exposure. Although UN operations can be ineffective or even damaging, as attested by the situation in Haiti, they can also be a useful – or the only – option for addressing humanitarian crises. Member states would likely be far less willing to approve UN field activities if they were vulnerable to significant financial risk. Despite frequent mismanagement and often-dubious results, there is little doubt that UN paralysis would result in suffering in some instances where it might otherwise be mitigated (Schaefer, 2013).

The UN's international responsibility takes place only on a voluntary basis and usually in the form of the payment of compensation. Moreover, none of the international legal bodies has jurisdiction over the UN owing to its immunity. This is an important factor for the realization of responsibility only after the voluntary acknowledgement of its fault by the UN. For example, after the UN operation in Congo in 1960s several states asked for compensation for harm, and the UN made agreements to make such payments (with Congo in 1961 and with Belgium in 1965). However, such a voluntary acknowledgement is incredibly rare.

In conclusion, it is possible to state that the issues of international responsibility for the spread of epidemics, pandemics and mass diseases are currently only generally regulated. The existing draft articles on responsibility of states and international organizations only points out the basic principle of the necessity to compensate the harm. However, practice shows that the subjects of international law in the majority of cases do not carry any international responsibility at all, and states like the Republic of Guinea or Haiti need more practical humanitarian help than legal regulation of their possible responsibility.

References

Amador, G. 1957. International responsibility. In United Nations (ed.) *Yearbook of the International Law Commission*, Volume II . New York: United Nations Publications, 173–231.

Ago, R. 1969. Review of previous work on codification of the topic of the international responsibility of states. In: *International Law Commission Yearbook* 2. New York: United Nations.

Carella, G. 1985. *La responsabilita dello Stato per crimini internazionali*. Bari: Jovene.

Caron, D. D. 1998. The basis of responsibility: attribution and other trans-substantive rules. In R. B. Lillich and D. B. Magraw (eds) *The Iran-United States Claims Tribunal: Its Contribution to the Law of State Responsibility*. New York: Transnational.

Crawford, J. 2002. *The International Law Commission's Articles on State Responsibility: Introduction, Text and Commentaries*. Cambridge: Cambridge University Press.

Criddle, E. J., Fox-Decent, E. A. 2008. Fiduciary theory of jus cogens. *The Yale Journal of International Law*, 34, 331–387.

Dupuy, P.-M. 1990. The international law of state responsibility: revolution or evolution? *Michigan Journal of International Law*, 1, 139–148.

Dupuy, P.-M. 1999. Reviewing the difficulties of codification on Ago's classification of obligations of means and obligations of result in relation to state responsibility. *European Journal of International Law*, 2, 371–385.

Greafrath. 1993. *Responsibility of States*. Thessaloniki: Institute of International Public Law and International Relations.

Knox, R. 2013. *Haitian Cholera Strain Spreads to Mexico*. NPR, 23 October 2013. Available online at www.npr.org/blogs/health/2013/10/23/239803890/haitian-cholera-strain-spreads-to-mainland-with-mexico-outbreak (accessed 26 October 2016).

Hsiung, J. C. 2004. *Anarchy, Hierarchy, and Actio Popularis: An International Governance Perspective*. The International Studies Association Annual Meeting, Montreal, Canada.

Office of the High Commissioner for Human Rights. 2000. CESCR General Comment (14: The Right to the Highest Attainable Standard of Health (Art. 12)). Available online at www.refworld.org/pdfid/4538838d0.pdf (accessed 26 October 2016).

Pellet, A. 2010. The definition of responsibility in international law. In J. Crawford, A. Pellet and S. Olleson (eds) *The Law of International Responsibility*. Oxford: Oxford University Press.

Reuter, P. 1995. *Le développement de l'ordre juridique international*. Paris: Economica.

Schaefer, B. D. 2013. *Haiti Cholera Lawsuit Against the U.N.: Recommendations for U.S. Policy*. Backgrounder No 2859. Available online at www.heritage.org/research/reports/2013/11/haiti-cholera-lawsuit-against-the-un-recommendations-for-us-policy (accessed 26 October 2016).

Transnational Development Clinic, Jerome N. Frank Legal Services Organization Yale Law School, Global Health Justice Partnership of the Yale Law School and the Yale School of Public Health, and Association Haïtienne de Droit de L'Environnment. 2013. *Peacekeeping without Accountability. The United Nations' Responsibility for the Haitian Cholera Epidemic*. Available online at www.law.yale.edu/documents/pdf/Clinics/Haiti_TDC_Final_Report.pdf (accessed 26 October 2016).

United Nations. 1959. *Yearbook of the International Law Commission*. Volume 1. New York, NY: United Nations Publications.

United Nations. 1966. International Covenant on Economic, Social and Cultural Rights. Adopted by General Assembly Resolution 2200 (XXI) of 16 December 1966. Available online at www.un-documents.net/icescr.htm (accessed on 26 October 2016).

UN News Center. 2014a. *Ban Issues 'International Rescue Call' to Halt Ebola Epidemic*. 5 September. Available online at www.un.org/apps/news/story.asp?NewsId=48651 (accessed 26 October 2016).

UN News Center. 2014b. *UN Chief to Leaders: 'The World Can and Must Stop Ebola – Now'*. 25 September 2014. Available online at www.un.org/apps/news/story.asp?NewsID=48852 (accessed 26 October 2016).

Vabres, D. 1947. Le jugement de Nuremberg et le principe de légalité des délits et des peines. *Revue de Droit Pénal et de Criminologie*, 10, 813–833.

Vitta, E. 1953. *Responsabilita Internazionale dello Stato per Atti Legislativi*. Milan: A. Giuffrè.

World Health Organization. 2003a. *Cumulative Number of Reported Probable Cases of Severe Acute Respiratory Syndrome*. Geneva: WHO. Available online at www.who.int/csr/sarscountry/2003_04_15/en/ (accessed 26 October 2016).

World Health Organization. 2003b. *Information to Member States Regarding Goods and Animals Arriving from SARS-Affected Areas*. Geneva: WHO. Available online at www. who.int/csr/sars/goods2003_04_10/en/ (accessed 26 October 2016).

World Health Organization. 2005. *International Health Regulations*, 2nd edn. Geneva: WHO. Available online at www.who.int/ihr/IHR_2005_en.pdf (accessed 26 October 2016).

3 Between ignorance, misperception and dilemma

Taking an ethical, epidemiological, and strategic look at crisis management during the 2014–15 Ebola outbreak in Liberia

Christian Janke

Introduction

In clinical medicine, the term 'crisis' tends to be perceived differently from its colloquial use. Here, it lacks the almost exclusively negative, apocalyptic connotation it bears in everyday language. Instead, the high development potential during a crisis is recognised, and the probability of attaining a new equilibrium as a result is understood both as a risk and an opportunity. The Ebola outbreak in West Africa, which is not over at the time of writing, has caused more than 11,000 deaths, the disruption of families, the suffering of survivors, countless orphans and a compromised health system and will no doubt lead to unpredictable medium- to long-term psychological, economic and political consequences. It above all appears to be a disaster the impact of which has still not been fully comprehended and hence a crisis, in the conventional sense of the term, that rumbles on. Why did international support take so long to come, and why was it performed so cumbersomely and hesitantly? Why did an outbreak of such magnitude hit almost everyone involved in an unprepared state? Why were the scarce resources allocated with so little thought given to actual needs for such a long time? Why were common sense and rationality, so often the first or at least the second victim of the outbreak? Answering these questions above all requires an analysis of misguided perceptions, assumptions and models.

This chapter is based on the experiences of the German humanitarian emergency relief in Liberia during the outbreak of Ebola in 2014–15, and in particular focuses on the lessons learnt in a close call that the German relief mission encountered within the crisis itself. For by the time the Ebola Treatment Unit (ETU) of the German Red Cross (DRK) and Federal Army Joint Support Mission was officially opened at the SKD Stadium in Monrovia on 23 December 2014, three months had already passed since the German defence minister had assigned the mission. There are valid reasons for a delay but none of them excuses the fact that taking three months to make an 'emergency response operation' operational is far too long. By the time the ETU was opened, it was no longer needed. The mission was about to be operationally terminated before it had even properly started working. How could this happen?

From global health to global health security

In August 2014, when the World Health Organization (WHO) declared the outbreak a 'public health emergency of international concern', the world was unsurprised and unmoved. Far more dramatic language was then used when on 18 September 2014 the United Nations Security Council called the outbreak a 'threat to the peace and security' and asked member states for robust counteractions. For global security providers like NATO searching for a justification to act in this unfamiliar situation this could have been the wake-up call. In reality, NATO remained asleep but some nations did heed the alarm. Only five days later, for example, the German defence minister took the bold and incisive decision to deploy a humanitarian Ebola relief mission of the German Armed Forces. With a lack of trained and dedicated troops, this Bundeswehr mission had to rely on volunteers and could only be realized in cooperation with the German Red Cross. Since then in Germany, as well as other countries, the role of the armed forces in such a scenario has been widely discussed. Facing the prospect of countless Ebola victims and an ongoing uncontrolled spread, even NGOs, who traditionally objected to cooperation with armed forces, began asking for military support. Undoubtedly, there is a strong association between conflict and health, however the causal chain is usually seen as going from a conflict to a compromised public health situation. Gro Harlem Brundtland, the former Norwegian prime minister and former secretary-general of the WHO, said in 2002:

> What if an outbreak takes place in a devastated Central African country where there is no local health care? What if security situation was so bad that we could not send in international experts to advise and assist in containing the outbreak? What if infected people start to flee into cities, to neighbouring countries and eventually out of the region?
>
> (Brundtland, 2002)

The spread of Ebola in Liberia and Sierra Leone, two post-civil war countries with devastated public services, painfully illustrate the accuracy of her prediction. Even worse, the association between conflict and health does not appear to be a one-way track (Fidler, 2005). What if an outbreak of a certain size and impact destabilizes a country or a region up to the point of failure of the state, riots and civil war? These were realistic scenarios for Ebola-affected countries in the West African region in September 2014 but Western armed forces' decision makers still found it difficult to consider the outbreak a security issue. After the orders of the German minister of defence were given there was more than a tendency among the leaders of the German Armed Forces Joint Medical Service to object to the commander's intent on the basis that they were unprepared for such a mission and refused to accept that the outbreak constituted a major security risk. This might partially explain why it took exactly another three months before the Ebola Treatment Unit of the German mission in Monrovia was finally operational on 23 December 2014. However, by this time 1,440 Ebola treatment beds were already available and there were only 66 Ebola patients left.

'Essentially, all models are wrong, but some are useful'

1440 ETU beds for 66 Ebola patients? In a country whose health sector lacks just about everything? Obviously, in a particular field of outbreak management, what is known as case management, massive overcapacities had developed that were not corrected. How could this have happened? As a rule, decision-making under uncertainty is based on explicit model assumptions. Not only were decisions concerning the distribution of scarce resources taken on the basis of these models, but cross-border traffic and, in some cases, even people's civil rights were restricted. A model published by the Centers for Disease Control and Prevention of the US Department of Health and Human Services in September 2014 forecast 1.4 million incidents of Ebola in Liberia and Sierra Leone for mid-January 2015 as an extreme case and a doubling of cases every 15 to 20 days (Meltzer *et al.*, 2014). In retrospect, it is now known that such a horrific scenario didn't occur. Should the inadequate models be blamed for the failures in allocation? Is the attempt to mathematically establish and forecast such complex developments a vain effort in any case?

It is true that the vast majority of models did not do justice to the complexity of events. For example, the epidemiologists underestimated the distinct effect of behavioural adaptation among key groups of the population (burial rites, no-touch policy). Perhaps an anthropologist should have helped the epidemiologists with modelling. What makes things even more complicated is that, as a rule, attempts at modelling take place far away from the epicentre, at universities in the Western world, which means that immediate 'situational awareness' of outbreak events is lost. Even so, effective outbreak management is inconceivable without suitable epidemiological models. The methods required for this purpose and specialist knowhow in the areas concerned are scattered across a wide range of subject fields. Here, innovative field epidemiologists without reservations towards other fields of science concerned are needed.

The obviously uncritical adoption of the models by the decision makers or their reluctance to adequately and immediately respond to clear discrepancies between theory and practice was at least just as problematic. Other NGOs and GOs in the immediate vicinity of the still-incomplete German facilities commenced operations although the numbers of incidents were successively dropping. Whereas the dynamics of events would have necessitated a daily review of one's own options to act, the 'inertia of masses', as well as a partly inflexible central steering of Germany's relief mission, resulted in a delay of the required adaptive efforts. But by New Year's Eve 2014 at the latest, as things stood, and following talks with national and international coordinators of Liberian outbreak management, it had become unequivocally clear that, in its classical configuration, Germany's ETU was not going to admit a single patient.

Disaster ethics between ignorance and dilemma

What would be even worse for a relief mission than its mere irrelevance would be the violation of the 'do not harm' principle, the *primum non nocere* of medical ethics. Just how easily one can fail to meet this requirement becomes apparent if one sets out from two relatively self-evident premises. First, Ebola patients ought to be treated in an isolated treatment unit. Second, non-Ebola patients should not be treated in such a unit (see Figure 3.1). The illustration shows the standardized layout of an isolated treatment unit. This is the configuration that was also used during the latest outbreak in Guinea, Sierra Leone and Liberia.

An isolated treatment unit of this kind provides neither individual nor sex-specific isolation. Suspected cases are initially merely allocated either to the 'Suspect Cases Area' or the 'Probable Case Area', depending on their assumed risk of infection. As soon as the infection is confirmed via molecular biological virus identification, patients are transferred to the 'Confirmed Positives Area'. In each of these areas, the non-Ebola patient bears a real, albeit differently high, risk of coming into contact with the virus and becoming infected within the treatment unit. In September and October 2014, precisely at the apex of the outbreak curve, most of the international organizations were intensifying their relief activities in West Africa, and Germany's humanitarian mission was conducting its first explorative exercise in Monrovia. At this time, a suspected case showing fever and other symptoms bore a high probability of then really being infected. Up to nine out of 10 suspected patients were subsequently confirmed by laboratory analysis; conversely, one out of every 10 patients was in the wrong

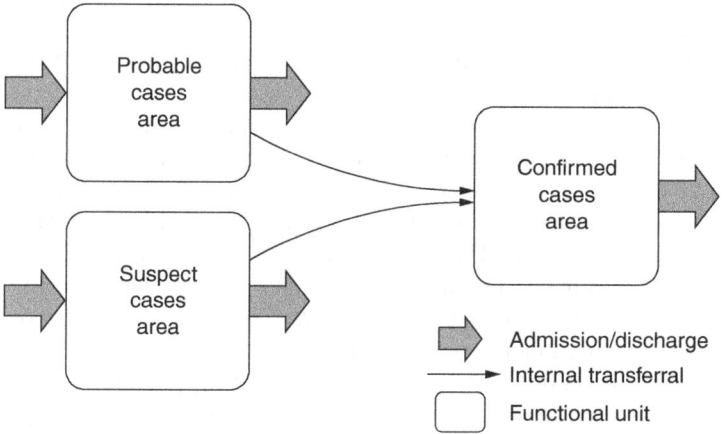

Figure 3.1 The conventional setting of an Ebola treatment unit.

treatment unit, in other words in one of the most dangerous places in the world. The only acceptable justification for this is the crisis situation and the complete lack of all necessary medical resources.

By January 2015, the incidences of the disease in Liberia had dropped significantly. However, as a result of the ETU isolation procedure, nine non-Ebola patients were now among the 10 suspected patients admitted to the ETUs. The Ebola case definition adopted by the WHO circumscribes a complex range of symptoms that occurs with a high probability when the disease is contracted. However, the probability of a symptom – like fever (or a symptom complex like the WHO case definition of EVD) occurring in Ebola is not at all identical with the probability of a patient showing this symptom complex having contracted Ebola. In other words, the probability that Santa Claus has a beard is unequal to the probability that somebody with a beard is Santa Claus. This mathematical phenomenon and, as a result, the lack of a reliable ETU admission criterion were widely ignored. In the three countries worst affected, this meant that by the end of December 2014 the overwhelming majority of the patients in the ETUs who were suffering from other diseases were now at risk of acquiring an Ebola virus infection in the treatment units. It therefore became increasingly irrational for a patient with symptoms typical of Ebola to consult an ETU. Large numbers of suspected patients fled Monrovia, and the epidemiological need to isolate, if possible, all suspected patients was severely compromised. Outbreak management in the field of Ebola case management was now in crisis itself (Lado *et al.*, 2015).

During the first few days of 2015, the officials of the German isolation unit in in Monrovia sought to devise a new strategy for their excellently trained and highly motivated Liberian and German specialists and for their sophisticated isolation treatment unit. At this point the issue of comprehensively optimizing Ebola case management was considered internally for the first time. Suspected patients were no longer to be separated merely corresponding to their risk of infection but also according to the probability of them not being infected. In addition to the three Suspect, Probable and Confirmed Positives Areas described above, two further separate areas, an Unlikely Cases Area and a Confirmed Negatives Area were required (see Figure 3.2).

Since there was an abundance of conventional ETUs in the immediate vicinity of the German one, the German relief mission was able to concentrate mainly on the two complementary areas, meaning that the ETU subsequently consisted of a Suspect Cases Area (already existent), an Unlikely Cases Area and a Confirmed Negatives Area. The ultimate objective was to avoid Ebola infections within the treatment unit at all costs. This is why the patients' freedom of movement in the Suspect Cases Area was confined to an approximately 2×3 m individual treatment compartment for the short period until the submission of the first laboratory result (4 to 12 hours). Patients testing positive for Ebola could be transferred to a conventional ETU, while those with negative results were immediately brought to the separate Unlikely Cases Area. Although an Ebola infection was not ruled out with absolute certainty with

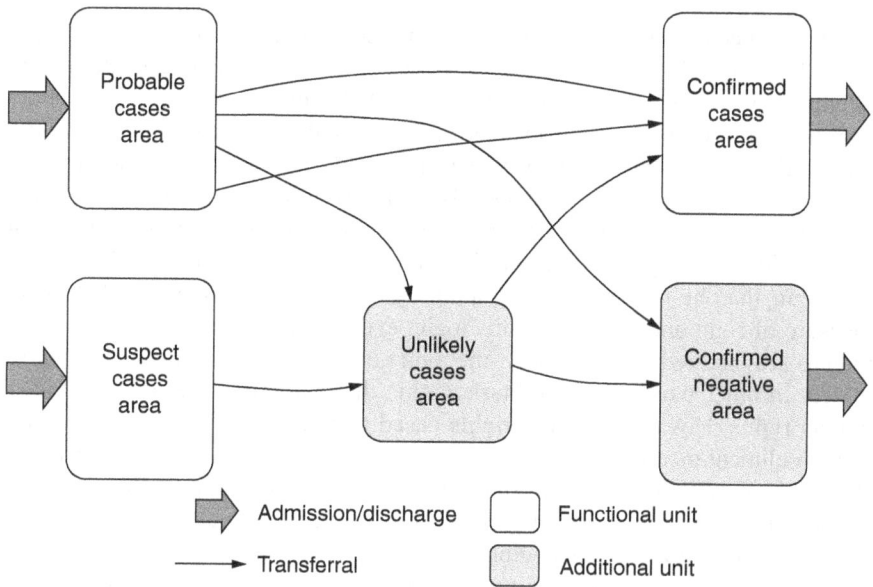

Figure 3.2 Structural adaptions of an Ebola treatment unit as suggested by the German humanitarian mission in West Africa in January 2015.

these patients, the risk of infectiousness for fellow patients was already approaching zero. Seventy-two hours after admission, with a negative lab result, Ebola could be ruled out with certainty, and transfer to the Confirmed Negatives Area was authorized. Here, the world now changed for the patients and those treating them. Much more time could be devoted to the individual patients, since staff no longer had to work in full protective gear. Above all, it was now possible to diagnose other diseases and offer causal treatment as well. This new type of an Ebola isolation facility was referred to as a Severe Infection Temporary Treatment Unit (SITTU). Relatively straightforward adjustments in terms of infrastructure and procedural organization effectively warded off a serious ethical and epidemiological problem. While ethical ignorance could thus be reduced, ethical dilemmas could not. Isolation treatment of Ebola suspects (as well as other aspects of Ebola outbreak management such as the quarantine of contact cases) will always be prone to the conflict between utilitarian and humanitarian schools of thought. Whereas the former demands an uncompromising isolation of possible cases (or even contact cases) for the sake of public protection, the latter insists on safeguarding individual human rights ('man is the measure of all things'). During outbreak management in a resource-poor country a trade-off between the two is necessary. For the decision makers on site, the dilemma had to be tolerated and could be measured in the unit 'number of nights sleep lost'.

A conceptual frame of outbreak response ethics

Much has been said and written about the Ebola outbreak in West Africa in 2014–15. Surprisingly incomplete, however, is the understanding of the ethical dilemmas involved. This chapter argues that, by examining the many short-comings and controversial decisions in Ebola outbreak management, the different ethical schools of thought which informed the practical decision-making should be attempted to be reconciled. But what were the most influential ethical theories at stake? Quarantine and triage, two key concepts of outbreak response interventions, clearly draw upon utilitarianism. They follow Jeremy Bentham's paradigm that 'it is the greatest happiness of the greatest number that is the measure of right and wrong'. In this logic, even extreme measures against individuals are justified if, in this way, the total utility for a population can be maximized. In other words, for a utilitarian ethic there are no inalienable individual human rights. However, such a 'rights-based approach' is the explicit principle of both clinical medicine and the work of many non-governmental organizations (NGOs) involved in the management of complex emergencies. Thus, for outbreak response missions the antithesis to utilitarianism is a humanist ethic.

During the 2014–15 Ebola outbreak in West Africa, many of the conflicts that took place can be conceptualized as clashes between these two ethical concepts. An extreme example was the plan to form a military cordon around the entire region affected in West Africa, a gigantic cordon sanitaire, which was accepted at least as a map exercise. The same principles, now put into practice, apply to the West Point intervention: in the wake of rioting and looting of an Ebola treatment unit, the Liberian government decided on 19 September 2014 to cordon off this township in the capital and prescribe a mass quarantine for its 75,000 inhabitants, which was maintained with the aid of firearms for 11 days. These measures follow a utilitarian logic, even though the two examples above, being neither balanced nor effective, could also be considered an epidemiological and ethical disaster. However, the underlying ethical dilemma has its roots in the fundamental decisions about the type and extent of isolation and quarantine. The clinical isolation regimes described in the last paragraph are not accepted as standard treatment of highly infectious diseases in the developed world. Cohort isolation is the domain of low-resource settings and, in its geographical determination, an expression of an unbalanced global distribution of resources and power. But why did all stakeholders stick to extremely substandard isolation policies for a region in Sub-Saharan Africa even after there was no longer a lack of medical resources by the end of 2014? Mowles observes that 'it is a particularly troubling development that organisations with an explicit moral mission to counter injustice and to encourage marginalised … groups to give voice to their needs, should adopt so uncritically (rationalist managerial) methods' (Mowles, 2010).

Theoretically, it is the medical sciences that could act as a role model for coping with this kind of ethical dilemma since the respective concepts are somewhat attached to different academic disciplines. Whereas public health ethics are often informed by utilitarian ideas, (clinical) medicine is still a stronghold of humanist ethics.

Lessons learnt?

None of the phenomena described here can be fully eliminated from crisis management, even if the underlying mechanisms are largely known.

In a complex emergency, it is impossible to completely abstain from managerial or, better, utilitarian approaches. This chapter has therefore argued for a hybridization and reconciliation of humanist and utilitarian strategies. This is not to say that the underlying conflicts, or the ethical dilemmas, can be completely dissolved. Adaptive strategic thinking is a key capacity for such a hybridization and, consequently, for 'good' management in complex emergencies and possibly beyond.

The global crises of the twenty-first century are characterized by unprecedented complexity, proximity and dynamics, and, in this regard, the 2014–15 Ebola outbreak in West Africa was certainly no exception. Even though insights and analyses exist, we have every reason for concern that on the next occasion we will again stumble over the ethical tripwires described and analysed above.

References

Bentham J. 1838–1843. *'The Works of Jeremy Bentham', published under the Superintendence of his Executor, John Bowring.* Edinburgh: William Tait. 11 vols. Vol. 4. Available at http://oll.libertyfund.org/titles/1925 (accessed 28 September 2016).

Brundtland, G. H. 2002. *Failed States and Global Security: How Health Can Contribute to a Safer World.* A Brookings Leadership Forum Address, 26 September 2002. Available online at www.brookings.edu/~/media/events/2002/9/26global-health/20020926. pdf (accessed 15 February 2016).

Fidler, D. P. 2005. Health as foreign policy: between principle and power. *Whitehead Journal of Diplomacy and International Relations*, 6, 179–194.

Lado, M., Walker, N. F., Baker, P., Haroon, S., Brown, C. S., Youkee, D., Studd, N., Kessete, Q., Maini, R., Boyles, T., Hanciles, E., Wurie, A., Kamara, T. B., Johnson, O. and Leather, A. J. M. 2015. Clinical features of patients isolated for suspected Ebola virus disease at Connaught Hospital, Freetown, Sierra Leone: a retrospective cohort study. *Lancet Infectious Diseases*, 15(9), 1024. Available online at www.ncbi.nlm.nih. gov/pubmed/26213248 (accessed 15 February 2016).

Meltzer, M. I., Atkins, C. Y., Santibanez, S., Knust, B., Petersen, B. W., Ervin, E. D., Nichol, S. T., Damon, I. K. and Washington, M. L. 2014. Estimating the future number of cases in the Ebola epidemic – Liberia and Sierra Leone, 2014–15. *CDC Morbidity and Mortality Weekly Report*, 63. Available online at www.cdc.gov/mmwr/pdf/other/ su6303.pdf (accessed 15 February 2016).

Mowles, C. 2010. Post-foundational development management – power, politics and complexity. *Public Administration and Development*, 30, 149–158.

4 The Canadian Armed Forces and their role in the Canadian response to the Ebola epidemic

Ethical and moral issues that guided policy decisions

Paul Eagan

The Ebola epidemic in West Africa has had a profound effect on Canadians and the world community. Its potential spread to Canada resulted in a domestic response that built upon the lessons learned from the Severe Acute Respiratory Syndrome (SARS) epidemic a decade previously. Internationally, Canada grappled with how best to contribute to the world effort to stem the outbreak. From the early stages of the epidemic, the Canadian government provided equipment, financial support, and laboratory expertise to the affected region. Initially, nongovernmental organizations provided clinical resources that were eventually overwhelmed and a request for military medical assistance was made.

This chapter reviews the whole of government response with particular reference to that of the Canadian Armed Forces (CAF). CAF worked with the British military to provide direct medical care in West Africa to health care workers who became infected with Ebola. To offer additional protection and treatment, an unproven, experimental Canadian vaccine was made available to military medical personnel in the event of a significant Ebola exposure. This chapter examines the Canadian response to the Ebola epidemic, including the ethical issues and dilemmas that informed policy decisions. These include the role of the military as a provider of humanitarian assistance, the allocation of scarce medical resources, the use of experimental vaccines in situations such as epidemics, and the CAF approach to the use of quarantine as a mechanism to control disease spread.

Introduction

The Canadian government made significant contributions to the global effort to control Ebola (Public Health Agency of Canada, 2015). Through financial assistance, donations of much-needed personal protective equipment, the provision of mobile labs to speed the diagnosis of Ebola, and providing promising vaccines to the WHO, the Canadian government and its agencies had a positive effect both at home and abroad. The painful lessons that were learned during the SARS outbreak have guided Canadian government priorities and capabilities over the last decade. The establishment of a more robust public health agency and a centralized laboratory and research institution, and the development of stronger cooperation at the federal and provincial level have better prepared Canada to manage domestic public health threats.

One of the government's key agencies has been the CAF. Although the CAF did not have a major role domestically, it played an important role in the government's international activities. This support included rapid transport of needed supplies and personnel to Sierra Leone as well as a medical mission called OP SIRONA (DND/Canadian Armed Forces, 2015).

Constrained resources—how to do more with less

The involvement of the CAF in the Canadian government Ebola response is one that consisted of some logistical challenges, as well as ethical decisions by the senior leadership. In a resource-constrained, military medical corps such as the CAF possesses, the question was asked as to whether it has the capability and depth of expertise to meet the challenge that the government requested. The principal concerns of Canadian civilian and military leaders were how best the Canadian military medical system could provide an effective and sustainable medical response to this humanitarian crisis (Bernier, 2015). The Canadian military medical system as it currently exists is not equipped to provide a sustainable medical capability in dealing with an epidemic such as Ebola. Much of its medical energies and expertise exist in the areas of short-term, emergency aid following natural disasters through a multidisciplinary unit, called the Disaster Assistance Response Team (DART) (DND/CAF, 2016). The DART mandate is to provide emergency support for up to 40 days until national and other international aid agencies are in place to provide long-term assistance. Providing a long-term humanitarian response to an infectious disease crisis was beyond the capability of the Canadian military health care system. The lack of a large pool of medical personnel made it essentially impossible for the Canadian military to provide a sustained response. It was estimated that if the Canadian military took over one of the 100-bed hospitals that were constructed by the United Kingdom in Sierra Leone it would have to effectively shut down its domestic medical capability and even then could only sustain a facility for approximately two months (Bernier, 2015). Not only was this not sustainable but this would also deny Canadian military members of an effective health care capability for domestic needs and deployed operations around the world. This was an untenable option.

There were additional concerns over the nature of the medical response and whether there existed sufficient expertise to provide an effective medical force, one that was capable of caring for seriously ill patients in a hospital setting. Presently, the CAF relies heavily on the Canadian civilian health care system to provide in-hospital care for its military members. Decisions made in the 1990s resulted in a significant downsizing of military hospitals and their eventual closure. Military physicians, nurses, and other health care professionals were dramatically decreased in number and those that remained were embedded in civilian hospitals across the country, where they could continue to provide some medical care to military members but also be in an environment where they could maintain their clinical skills and expertise.

These various skills and expertise in critical care nursing, internal medicine, infectious diseases, and in-hospital care are the very skills required for a humanitarian medical mission to West Africa. It became apparent that if the CAF medical system were going to provide some assistance in West Africa it would have to be as part of a joint effort with one of its allies and in a targeted way that could effectively make the most difference to the people of Sierra Leone.

This led to discussions and consultations at various levels of government between its major allies, which included the United States, France, and the United Kingdom (Bernier, 2015). What eventually transpired was a decision to work with the United Kingdom's Defence Medical Services and aid their efforts to staff and provide high-quality medical care and expertise to ill health care providers (both indigenous and international NGOs) in Sierra Leone (DND/Canadian Armed Forces, 2015).

One of the major difficulties in the fight against Ebola in West Africa was the devastating effect of Ebola on perhaps the scarcest of resources in Sierra Leone: the medical expertise and health care providers in the country (Evans et al., 2015). The very people who could help turn the tide against this epidemic were themselves at high risk of becoming infected and dying. As well, civilian health care professionals working with NGOs are more likely to come to work at Ebola treatment centres if they are comfortable with the knowledge that high-quality medical care is readily available to them should they become ill. Embedding a Canadian contingent with the UK medical effort (UK Ministry of Defence, 2015) not only helped the British military medical system and its mission but also allowed Canada to contribute in a positive and sustained manner that would have the most dramatic and long-lasting effect.

Health care workers—does Canadian society and the military owe a higher level of care and responsibility?

One of the many ethical dilemmas that informed the decision-making processes for the CAF response is the question of society's responsibility to health care workers that it sends into harm's way. In this case, it is not bullets or armed combat that puts them at risk, but instead the invisible but real risk of contracting and potentially dying of a fatal illness. Although CAF military health care workers eagerly volunteered for the mission, the act of volunteerism does not abrogate or dismiss the societal and institutional responsibility to protect these altruistic workers to the best of society's and the organization's capabilities. Since these health care workers are at a far greater risk of acquiring Ebola because of where they are going and the patient population that they are treating, they require at least if not a greater level of training and support as those who remain at home to treat possible, but less likely to occur domestic Ebola cases. Within the literature on medical ethics, public health ethics and professional medical obligations, there is much discussion regarding physicians' duty to treat and a corresponding duty to ensure those providing treatment have adequate protection against infectious disease This is often known as the value of reciprocity. According to many medical ethicists, is a societal obligation and the most ethically correct choice (Singer et al., 2003; Brody and Avery, 2009).

In the context of the Canadian military and making the necessary operational choices and commitments, this means that there is an obligation to assure that CAF health care workers have access to the same level of care as civilian Canadian health care workers and in a similar timely fashion. They are also entitled to specific training and personal protective equipment to make sure that they can perform their duties in as safe a manner as possible. This includes access to prophylaxis and treatment. The question is how does one do this halfway around the world from Canada? How do you do this in a country such as Sierra Leone, which lacks the necessary capability and resources? There is also the dilemma that if the already-scarce resources that exist in West Africa are diverted to care for Canadians, then these resources are not available to the local population and its health care workers, both indigenous and those working with NGOs. The answers to these ethical problems were approached in a stepwise fashion, the first being the issue of air evacuation capability.

To assure that there was an adequate aeromedical evacuation capability that could effectively and quickly return CAF medical health care providers home to access specialized care at one of the designated Ebola treatment centres in Canada was the priority. In the fall of 2014, there was essentially no one in either the civilian or military sector that could provide a robust aeromedical capability from Africa to Canada. The unique requirements included an aircraft that is capable of flying nonstop from West Africa to Canada. This impediment had already been identified by the limited number of civilian carriers who describe the almost insurmountable issues of obtaining overflight rights and landing privileges for refuelling when they tried to transport Ebola-positive patients back to the United States or Europe (International SOS, 2014). The Canadian military is fortunate in that it does have transport planes that are capable of this long flight, although owing to limited numbers of aircraft and the heavy demands on them to support military operations the availability of these aircraft is problematic and in particular during these crisis and time sensitive situations where transport of Ebola-infected patients is required in just a few days. On top of that is the necessity of providing a high level of protection to the flight crew and medical staff providing care while in transit.

The Canadian military had got rid of its Cold War era air transport isolation chamber in the 1990s, and so a novel approach was developed as a stopgap measure. It consisted of using a specially designed ambulance, which had been designed for the transport of chemical and biological warfare casualties, and repurposing it for aerovac purposes as a drive-on negative pressure transport chamber (Clifford, 2014). Further development of temporary but durable antechambers for safe donning and doffing of PPE followed. After additional training of aerovac personnel in the use of the specialized PPE, the transport capability was deemed operational in November 2014.

Training of personnel was the next major issue that needed to be addressed. Although it was now only a dozen years since the SARS epidemic, the necessary practical training and expertise to train CAF health care professionals in the proper donning and doffing of personal protective equipment was difficult to obtain domestically. As mentioned previously, there was no in-house capability within the Canadian military. The UK military was approached and agreed to provide an extensive training program (DND/Canadian Armed Forces, 2015), which was currently being used by them to train their own military health care providers (UK Ministry of Defence, 2015). This training was also very beneficial as it led to a harmonization of standard operating procedures and approaches within the binational medical treatment team and helped contribute to team cohesion.

The Ebola vaccine—an untested treatment

Another ethical issue is that of the use of an untested vaccine against Ebola by Canadian military medical personnel. The experimental vaccine (Public Health Agency of Canada, 2014a) is a recombinant vesicular stomatitis virus-derived vaccine (VSV-EBOV) that had been developed by the National Microbiological Laboratory, which is part of the Public Health Agency of Canada. This vaccine had shown promising results in nonhuman primate studies, where it appeared to have a role as a prophylactic, preexposure vaccine as well as for immediate postexposure prophylaxis. However, the vaccine had never been tested in humans. As part of the government of Canada's response to the Ebola epidemic, it was announced in November 2014 that the Public Health Agency of Canada was going to work with Canadian research institutions as part of a Phase I clinical trial of this vaccine (Public Health Agency of Canada, 2014a). This would be held in conjunction with a similar trial in the United States and Europe that involved the WHO. As part of the clinical trial, the decision was made to make the vaccine available to civilian health care providers at all of the designated Ebola treatment centres across Canada as an immediate postexposure prophylaxis treatment. An extensive and detailed informed consent process was developed as part of the clinical trial.

Since the CAF have an ethical obligation to provide the same level of care to military health care providers as is provided in a domestic health care setting to civilian health care providers, it was felt that this vaccine should also be pre-positioned in Sierra Leone at the hospital where the Canadian military health care workers were working. This was particularly important as the senior leadership recognized that the military health care workers were in fact at greater risk of exposure to Ebola given the fact that they were working at the front lines of the Ebola epidemic (Bernier, 2015). However, there was significant protocol issues and problems for the Canadian military to be part of the Canadian-based

Phase I clinical trial. In the end, it was felt by the civilian director of the Canadian trial that CAF health care workers would not be eligible for this clinical trial (Bernier, 2015). There were, therefore, questions and concerns regarding how best to proceed in an ethically responsible manner. The decision was made to proceed with the procurement of the experimental vaccine directly from the Public Health Agency of Canada as part of the special access program (SAP), which allows the military to obtain medications and therapies that have not yet been formally approved for use in Canada. As this was an unapproved therapy that was now being considered outside of a clinical trial, it was felt to be critically important that an independent ethics review board should evaluate and assess the decision to not be part of a clinical trial while making the vaccine available to military health care workers through SAP (Veritas IRB, 2014).

To help frame the response, the review board was asked specific questions about the ethical arguments for and against the vaccine's use.

The first of these questions was whether it is ethical to offer the vaccine to a Canadian military member that has experienced a significant suspected or known exposure in what amounts to a compassionate use scenario. To answer this question, an analysis of the risk:benefit ratio associated with the use of this vaccine was done. On the risk side of the equation, the Ebola outbreak in West Africa had a reported case fatality rate of between 50 and 60 percent. Without any proven effective treatment options for Ebola, the only current available treatment was supportive therapy. The efficacy of the vaccine was unknown although the results of animal research were encouraging. At the time of this decision, the Phase I studies were just getting under way, and the vaccines efficacy remained unknown in humans. If it were known to be effective, engaging in additional clinical research trials would not be ethical as there would be no equipoise. The IRB felt that as the efficacy in humans was unknown so was the potential risk for harm. The preliminary data in both humans and animals had shown that the risk profile could outweigh the potential for benefit.

The IRB felt that given the comparative lack of data about the vaccine, a detailed and transparent consent process that covered all aspects of the vaccine and its proposed use was of critical importance when offering the vaccine to CAF members. The IRB felt that the detailed advanced briefing that was to be provided to CAF members prior to deployment to West Africa was excellent and critical to a truly informed consent process. They stressed that the consent process must provide straightforward information about risks, benefits, purpose, and most importantly the uncertainty pertaining to the vaccine (Veritas IRB, 2014). It was important that all efforts were made to avoid the potential misunderstanding that this drug had been proven to be efficacious and to ensure expectations, both good and bad, were appropriately managed. It was also important that this informed consent process/briefing needed to occur well in advance of any possible exposure, since once a potential breach of protective protocols occurred the vaccine needed to be administered within 30 minutes.

With respect to compassionate use, the board felt that a more appropriate term was "monitored emergency use" (Veritas IRB, 2014), as this term was better associated with a commitment to sharing clinical outcomes and knowledge with the broader community. With respect to the ethics of offering the vaccine not in the context of a research trial, there were concerns expressed about what the ramifications would be to the public broadly. Some board members felt that randomized controlled trials were necessary to prove the efficacy of the vaccine, which would eventually help the general population and not just the few individuals who gained access through the special access program. Other IRB members promoted the position that the collection of strong evidence about the vaccine was paramount and the compassionate use of the vaccine interfered with this concept. Still others argued that randomized control trials were ethically problematic when mortality was so high, and there was no standard of care that was truly effective. The most important objective was to get useful data, even if it is not through an RCT, which can be cumbersome and delay the release of critical clinical information, which may result in loss of life.

The research board felt that the October 2014 WHO report (WHO Ethics Working Group, 2014) on this issue was dated and the context in which it was written had changed over time as the epidemic rapidly progressed. Its guidance was no longer as valid since the outbreak was not contained and had affected tens of thousands of people around the world. The greater duty now was to ensure that vital research is carried out so that an approved vaccine would be available for a greater number of people, rather than a handful through special access programs and clinical trials. The IRB stressed that if special access programs were to be carried out, a strong commitment at a minimum must be made to share that knowledge (Veritas IRB, 2014). In addition, large SAPs were not ethical in the current context of the epidemic.

The crux of the issues concerning the ethical feasibility of using a drug through the SAP was the tension between the benefit to the individual versus that of the larger population. Since the mission of the military was to come to the assistance of others, there was likely a higher duty towards the greater good of the larger population as opposed to the duty to a select few.

The chief concern about SAPs was that they would adversely affect participation in formal clinical research trials. Research has the best potential to lead to more equitable and just health care provision than when rationed to individuals through SAP. In addition, research can prove efficacy, an important element to assure the broad distribution and approval of the vaccine.

Given the concerns with administering the vaccine through SAP, what makes it ethical to use it in this context? One benefit is that clinical information from SAPs could help fill the knowledge gaps that necessitate their existence. The more rapid production of evidence might either decrease the number of future patients who are harmed by interventions that are ultimately found to be unsafe or ineffective, or increase the number of future patients who could confidently access effective interventions (Walker et al., 2014). The risks and benefits of using unproven interventions for individuals faced with life-threatening illnesses differ considerably from those at a population level. Those individuals' attitudes towards the uncertainties and trade-offs in decisions when it comes to using unproven interventions are likely to be based on their unique circumstances. In such cases, looking for even a slight chance of improvement is a rational choice. Restricting access may increase suffering for those who feel that they have nothing to lose, whether or not the intervention works, and so may be considered to cause harm disproportionate to the potential harms that are arising. Compassion and the circumstances seemed to urge allowing access (Walker et al., 2014).

The conclusion of the IRB review was that, given the high rates of mortality in those infected with Ebola and the lack of approved treatment, the potential benefits of administering the investigational vaccine as a postexposure prophylaxis outweighed the potential risks. The recommendation for its use was with the understanding that the knowledge gained must be shared as broadly as possible. Also, continued efforts must be made to link with the research trial should more vaccine be made available to the CAF through the SAP. Additionally, CAF needs to consider other ethical issues associated with the distribution of the vaccine, specifically, how it would be rationed in the event of a shortage for CAF members (Veritas IRB, 2014).

The second question asked if it is unethical to not offer the vaccine to a CAF member who has experienced a significant suspected or known exposure. It was interesting that the IRB largely felt that if the vaccine were available through the program it would be unethical not to offer it to a CAF member (Veritas IRB, 2014). The principal reasons for this opinion included, first, that only a small number of vaccines are in fact made available to CAF, which means that it is not taking a significant number of vials away from the supply available for research. Second, since Ebola is an easily contracted and potentially fatal disease, offering the vaccine is important in such illnesses. This is in contrast to a chronic condition, where there is the opportunity to live and the possibility of a cure being found some time in the future. Third, the strong preliminary animal research that suggested a potential benefit makes the ethical decision of offering the vaccine easier. Finally, there is the duty to care principle, in which the Department of National Defence has an obligation to its CAF members to protect them over others as the CAF health care workers are putting their lives at risk for the benefit of their patients.

There was a dissenting view that it is not unethical not to offer the vaccine (Veritas IRB, 2014). Although the morbidity and mortality statistics for Ebola are serious, the efficacy of the vaccine remains unknown in humans. If the vaccine were proven to be efficacious, clinical trials would not be required. Given the lack of efficacy, the possible harm associated with the unproven vaccine, and debate about the ethics of even using the vaccine under SAP, it would not be unethical not to offer a vaccine with unknown efficacy and risks.

In closing, the opinion of the IRB was that the high mortality rate of individuals infected with Ebola and the decided lack of approved treatment beyond supportive care supported the potential benefits of administering the experimental vaccine for postexposure prophylaxis as these benefits outweighed the potential risks (Veritas IRB, 2014). Despite the fact that it was not part of a randomized controlled trial, it is important that any knowledge that is gained through the use of this vaccine under SAP access must be widely shared and that there should be an ongoing effort to link any usage of the vaccine by CAF with a research trial.

On the basis of this assessment, five and eventually a total of 10 vials of the experimental vaccine were positioned at the medical treatment facility in Sierra Leone where the Canadians worked and treated potentially Ebola-infected patients (Clifford, 2015). Over the course of the medical mission, there were no breaches of personal protective equipment or a needle-stick injury that required the consideration of vaccine usage.

Isolation or quarantine?

The final ethical consideration for discussion is the issue of quarantine or the softer term of self-isolation for military medical health care workers returning from Sierra Leone. The CAF mission to Sierra Leone represented the largest deployment of Canadian nationals to the Ebola-affected region, and guidance was required for when they returned to Canada. The development of recommendations by CAF with respect to postdeployment medical surveillance and management of travelers from Ebola endemic areas was informed in a number of different ways. The Public Health Agency of Canada (PHAC) develops general Canadian guidance, and it has been long-standing policy of the military to adhere to PHAC guidance whenever possible (Tepper, 2014). The federal guidance is informed by expert opinion and recommendations by the World Health Organization and the US Centers for Disease Control and Prevention. It is also guided by the Federal Quarantine Act (Government of Canada, 2005), which is in turn interpreted and enforced by provincial public health authorities. Unfortunately, the final quarantine and self-isolation policies are not always based on sound science but rather on perceived risk rather than real risk. As is often the case, there is a delicate balance that must be considered when individual rights and freedoms are at loggerheads with the public good. This was particularly an issue with Ebola, where the fear of Ebola spread led some public officials in the United States to impose quarantines on returning travelers, in spite of medical evidence and opinion to the contrary (Drazen et al., 2014).

The approach that was taken by the CAF drew from PHAC guidance (Public Health Agency of Canada, 2014b) and used a risk stratification matrix based on the presence or absence of Ebola-like symptoms at the time of return to Canada (Directorate of Force Health Protection, 2015). Asymptomatic travelers were further stratified based on the nature of their duties (e.g., whether they did or did not provide direct patient care) and whether there was a known breach of protocol while wearing personal protective equipment and providing care to Ebola-infected patients. If deemed at high risk of exposure, organized accommodation at a single location was available where asymptomatic, high-risk travelers could freely move while receiving appropriate medical care and follow-up. There was also the opportunity for those who were low-risk travelers to choose to self-isolate away from family to stay at the high-risk exposure location.

Over the course of the mission there were no high-risk exposures, and all returning CAF medical personnel were classified as low-risk exposure health care providers as per the risk matrix for postmission surveillance. As a result, they were all allowed to return to their homes, where they were on restricted duties that did not permit any patient care duties. They performed daily monitoring of body temperature and maintained a symptom log so that early signs of possible Ebola infection could be identified and reported to their health care provider. They were also advised to avoid large public gatherings. This was mostly for their personal protection as these venues are locations where their risk of exposure to upper respiratory tract infections and gastrointestinal diseases is high. Unfortunately, many of the symptoms of these common but benign conditions are similar to those of Ebola in its early stages and can confuse early patient management. CAF public health personnel also established a close working relationship with local public health officers to keep them informed and to seek their guidance when necessary.

In closing, the recent CAF involvement in the Canadian government response to the Ebola epidemic in West Africa resulted in a number of ethical issues that informed and guided the actions and the nature of the response. These ethical dilemmas are not specific to Ebola, and they have been considered previously in pandemic flu preparations, the SARS outbreak, and other similar public health events. As is so frequently said, failure to learn from the past often dooms one to repeat previous mistakes. The devastation that characterized the Ebola epidemic gives reason to reflect, remember, and learn so that one is better prepared for the next epidemic that will surely come.

References

Bernier, J. 2015. Interview, March 2015.

Brody, H. and Avery, E. N. 2009. Medicine's duty to treat pandemic illness: solidarity and vulnerability. *Hastings Center Report*, 39(1), 40–48.

Clifford, P. 2014. Interview, November 2014.

Clifford, P. 2015. Interview, April 2015.

Directorate of Force Health Protection. 2015. *Health Protection Recommendations for Deployment to West Africa in Support of Ebola Virus Disease Response: Post Mission Surveillance*. Ottawa: Department of National Defence, Canadian Armed Forces.

DND/CAF. 2016. *Disaster Assistance Response Team*. Available online at www.forces. gc.ca/en/operations-abroad-recurring/dart.page (accessed September 10, 2016).

DND/Canadian Armed Forces. 2015. *OP SIRONA*. Available online at www.forces.gc.ca/ en/operations-abroad/op-sirona.page (accessed September 10, 2016).

Drazen, J. M., Kanapathipillai, R., Campion, E. W., Rubin, E. J., Hammer, S. M., Morrissey, S. and Baden, L. R. 2014. Ebola and quarantine. *New England Journal of Medicine*, 371, 2029–2030.

Evans, D. K., Goldstein, M. P. and Popova, A. 2015. *The Next Wave of Deaths from Ebola? The Impact of Health Care Worker Mortality*. Policy research working paper no. WPS 7344. Washington, DC: World Bank. Available online at http://documents. worldbank.org/curated/en/408701468189853698/The-next-wave-of-deaths-from-Ebola-the-impact-of-health-care-worker-mortality (accessed September 10, 2016).

Government of Canada. 2005. Quarantine Act. Available online at http://laws-lois.justice.
gc.ca/eng/acts/Q-1.1/page-1.html (accessed September 11, 2016).

International SOS. 2014. *Evacuation of Doctors Exposed to Ebola in Sierra Leone*. Available online at www.internationalsos.com/case-studies/case-study-folder/evacuation-of-doctors-exposed-to-ebola-in-sierra-leone (accessed September 11, 2016).

Public Health Agency of Canada. 2014a. *Fact Sheet – VSV-EBOV – Canada's Experimental vaccine for Ebola*. Available online at www.canada.ca/en/public-health/services/infectious-diseases/fact-sheet-ebov-canada-s-experimental-vaccine-ebola.html (accessed August 10, 2017).

Public Health Agency of Canada. 2014b. *Interim Guidance: Public Health Management of Cases And Contacts of Human Illness Associated with Ebola Virus Disease*. Available online at www.canada.ca/en/public-health/services/diseases/ebola/health-professionals-ebola/interim-guidance-public-health-management-cases-contacts-ebola-community-setting-canada.html (accessed August 10, 2017).

Public Health Agency of Canada. 2015. *Canada's Response to Ebola*. Available online at www.healthycanadians.gc.ca/diseases-conditions-maladies-affections/disease-maladie/ebola/response-reponse/index-eng.php?id=response (accessed September 10, 2016).

Singer, P. A., Benatar, S. R., Bernstein, M. and Daar, A. S. 2003. Ethics and SARS: lessons from Toronto. *British Medical Journal*, 327(7427, December 6, 2003), 1342–1344.

Tepper, M. 2014. Interview, October 2014.

UK Ministry of Defence. 2015. *OP Gritrock*. Available online at www.army.mod.uk/agc/37140.aspx (accessed September 12, 2016).

Veritas IRB. 2014. *Use of a Recombinant Vesicular Stomatitis Virus Expressing the Envelope Glycoprotein of Ebola Virus Zaire (rVSV ZEBOV-GP) Vaccine for Post-Exposure Prophylaxis for Ebola Virus Exposure*. Montreal: Veritas IRB.

Walker, M. J., Rogers, W. A. and Entwistle, V. 2014. Ethical justifications for access to unapproved medical interventions: an argument for (limited) patient obligations. *American Journal of Bioethics*, 14(11), 3–15.

WHO Ethics Working Group. 2014. *Ethical Issues Related to Study Design for Trials on Therapeutics for Ebola Virus Disease*. Geneva: World Health Organization.

5 "If you let it get to you …"

Moral distress, ego-depletion, and mental health among military health care providers in deployed service

Jillian Horning, Lisa Schwartz, Matthew Hunt, and Bryn Williams-Jones

Introduction

Health care providers (HCPs) are routinely placed into morally challenging situations that have the potential to cause moral distress. This is especially true for HCPs working in the military, whether they are on deployment outside their typical contexts of practice such as in disaster relief (e.g., Haiti and the Ebola missions in West Africa), or in more typically military settings such as peacekeeping or armed conflicts (e.g., Afghanistan, Syria). Moral distress refers to "painful feelings and/or psychological disequilibrium" (Nilsson, Sjöberg, Kallenberg, and Larsson, 2011, p. 50) that occur when an individual is aware of a morally appropriate action in a moral dilemma but obstruction prevents them from carrying it out, or when in a situation where they must choose between upholding equally treasured but conflicting moral values. Similarly, moral distress can occur when faced with a "tragic choice" where all available courses of action require something of moral significance to be given up, such as surgical triage in a mass casualty event (Hunt, Sinding, and Schwartz, 2012). In the literature, moral distress has been connected to negative psychological effects and even stress-related mental health issues including compassion fatigue, burnout, and post-traumatic stress disorder (Owen and Wanzer, 2014; Gustafsson, Eriksson, Strandberg, and Norberg, 2010; Litz et al., 2009).

The most recent model of moral distress in military HCPs was created by Bradshaw and colleagues, who argue that the result of the cumulative effects of moral distress could lead to a crisis state for military HCP where they are no longer able to cope and maintain normal functioning (Bradshaw, Brajtman, Cragg, and Higuchi, 2010). Based on theories of stress in psychology, they propose the incorporation of a feedback loop to describe the observed cumulative effects of unresolved moral distress. The psychological mechanism underpinning this feedback loop and driving the cumulative progression of moral distress has been undiscussed in the literature. This chapter will describe military HCPs' experiences with the moral distress process and assess the potential use of "ego-depletion" as a psychological mechanism and conceptual framework for its cumulative progression. Since ego-depletion is caused by the over-taxing of limited self-regulation resources, the demands placed on these resources through-out the experience of moral distress are relevant here. If HCPs are unable to achieve satisfactory resolution, moral distress (especially when experienced chron-ically) can be associated with heightened personal resource demands and con-tinued ego-depletion, which creates a cycle towards mental health problems (Gao et al., 2014; Rivkin, Diestel, and Schmidt, 2015). The personal effects of this depletion can include depression, burnout and further difficulties the result of which are breakdowns in relationships, higher need for health care resources, and potentially loss of employment (Rivkin, Diestel, and Schmidt, 2015; Owen and Wanzer, 2014; Jones et al., 2008; McCarthy and Deady, 2008). For the military, this can have significant effects on personnel and resource management.

Methods

This chapter is based on data collected by the Ethics in Military Medicine Research Group (EMMRG) in a Canadian Institutes of Health Research-funded study examining the ethical challenges of military health care professionals during peacekeeping or disaster response missions, and exploring both their role with patients and their role within the mission, and how ethical tensions are addressed (www.emmrg.ca; Williams-Jones, de Laat, Rochon, Okhowat, Schwartz, and Horning, 2015). This study follows on from research by Schwartz, Hunt et al. that examined ethical challenges experienced by HCPs working in the context of humanitarian assistance and development work (Williams-Jones et al., 2015; Schwartz et al., 2010). Here we use the data to help understand how moral distress is experienced in distinctive ways in the military HCP population, and to represent this process by applying psychological theory to the research findings.

We used purposive sampling to identify potential participants from all types of health professions, with a variety of experiences, and who had spent at least six months between 2005 and 2010 working on medical missions in an inter-national context with the Canadian Armed Forces (CAF). The qualitative ana-lysis consists of 27 interviews of male and female non-civilian HCPs in the CAF, including nurses, physicians, assistants, medical technicians, and physio-therapists. Recruitment occurred in three stages: (1) invitations were mailed in English and French and 350 HCPs were given individual invitations to parti-cipate along with a letter of support from the Deputy Surgeon General; (2) snow-ball recruitment; (3) and contact through the research team via the EMMRG website as well as through advisory board members. Interviews using open-ended questions were conducted. The interview guide was created with the intention of prompting participants to discuss different aspects of their personal ethical experiences in the deployed context.

The first step of the analysis involved descriptive coding of EMMRG parti-cipant interviews and conducting a combined inductive and deductive approach to analysis (Miles and Huberman, 1994). The second step, described here, involved analysing EMMRG participant experiences through the lens of Bradshaw and colleagues' model using deductive coding and decision modeling and finally outlining emerging themes that challenged aspects of the model.

Bradshaw and colleagues' model was used as a lens to better understand the experience of moral distress in EMMRG participants' interviews and was selected as it is the most recent and fully developed model for military nurses, includes conceptualization of a resolution process, and incorporates findings from psychology including aspects of stress models. A secondary set of deductive codes were created that reflected Bradshaw and colleagues' model and its associated steps was combined with the general findings, and descriptive qualitative analysis was then used to develop themes relevant to the phenomenon of moral distress in military HCP.

Approach of analysis

1   Interviews conducted, anonymized, transcribed
2   Primary deductive coding hierarchy based on interview guide
3   Inductive incorporation of emerging themes into primary coding hierarchy
4   Secondary deductive coding hierarchy based on Bradshaw and colleagues' model
5   Inductive incorporation of emerging themes relevant to moral distress from primary coding hierarchy into secondary coding hierarchy
6   Descriptive qualitative analysis of secondary coding hierarchy

---

The type of "low-inference" interpretation in descriptive qualitative analysis captures the individual's meaning regarding their personal experiences with the phenomenon of moral distress (Sandelowski, 2000). This approach requires that the researcher interpret the language used by participants as a "vehicle of communication" to convey the facts of military HCPs' experiences with moral distress and the meaning that they associate with these facts (Sandelowski, 2000). The study was reviewed and approved by research ethics committees at the University of Montreal, McMaster University, and the Department of National Defence/CAF.

Background

Moral challenges for deployed military health care providers

Military service members frequently confront moral dilemmas during war (Gibbons, Shafer, Hickling, and Ramsey, 2013; Litz et al., 2009). For a military HCP, the dual role of healer and service member adds another dimension of moral complexity to practicing in the deployed environment (Gibbons et al., 2013). While military HCPs have a duty to care for their patients, they may encounter situations when the military mission is seen as primary and prioritized over patient needs, putting "health care providers in ethically compromising situations that leave lasting impressions" (Gibbons et al., 2013). The challenge of balancing military and professional moral values increases the likelihood of military HCPs encountering moral dilemmas (Gibbons et al., 2013). Fry and colleagues (2002) argue that military nurses work in diagnosis and treatment settings that are atypical and stressful. Stewart (2009) reports that military health care teams in the deployed environment regularly encounter horrific traumatic injuries and deaths, with 69 percent of cases involving polytrauma (Owen and Wanzer, 2014). A UK study examining military medical personnel found that providing care to combat trauma cases, witnessing soldiers being wounded or killed, and handling dead bodies was associated with psychological distress in medical personnel (Jones et al., 2008). Other sources of stress for military HCPs include separation from family and support systems, 24/7 availability, exposure to personal danger, friends and coworkers being injured or killed, and potentially being involved in killing (Adler and Castro, 2013; Jones et al., 2008).

Frequent moral challenges as well as highly stressful and complex patient care situations in the deployed environment present heightened risks for military HCPs to encounter both psychological and moral distress. Some research has been conducted on the impact of moral challenges on military HCPs' mental health, with Jones and colleagues (2008) suggesting that moral stressors contribute to the high levels of stress-related mental health problems in this population (Litz et al., 2009; Gibbons et al., 2013; Vargas, Hanson, Kraus, Drescher, and Foy, 2013; Dombo, Gray, and Earl, 2013). While there is limited research available, the concepts of both moral distress and, more recently, moral injury have been examined in military HCPs encountering moral dilemmas in the field (Fry, Harvey, Hurley, and Foley, 2002; Bradshaw et al., 2010; Gibbons et al., 2013).

Moral distress experience for deployed military HCPs

When military HCPs encounter a moral dilemma, they choose a course of action to pursue, that is, they make a "moral action choice" (MAC) (Bradshaw et al., 2010). This process involves awareness of the situation as conflicting with one's personal moral values, followed by an appraisal of the situation, and a moral judgement deciding on the best course of action given the context (Fry et al., 2002; Bradshaw et al., 2010). However, this process is lived out in frequently rushed and messy contexts and may be more reactive at the individual level. Furthermore, contextual factors in the deployed environment sometimes create barriers that prevent HCPs from enacting a desired MAC, forcing them to choose between upholding equally treasured moral values and presenting them with a tragic choice, leading to the experience of moral distress (Nilsson et al., 2011; Hunt, Sinding, and Schwartz, 2011).

Moral distress, moral injury, and psychological distress

In the literature, the concepts of moral injury and psychological distress are related to moral distress and contribute to better understanding the experiences of military HCPs. Both moral distress and moral injury reflect conceptually similar experiences; in contrast, though interconnected, psychological distress represents a distinct phenomenon (McCarthy and Deady, 2008). Psychological distress involves one's emotional reactions to a situation "but does not necessarily involve violation of core values and duties" (Epstein and Hamric, 2013, p. 331) as is experienced by those with moral distress (Litz et al., 2009). When a challenging situation involves a specifically moral dimension, an individual's existing moral standards, beliefs, and world views (moral schemas) are challenged in a way that is not necessarily experienced during psychological distress (Litz et al., 2009; Harding, 1985). Moral distress often involves psychological distress but also involves emotional and spiritual components that may alter a HCP's self-identity and beliefs that "the world is benevolent, the world is meaningful, and the self is worthy" (Litz et al., 2009, p. 698). As such, this chapter will use "psychological distress" when outlining nonmoral emotional reactions, and the term "moral distress" when discussing applicable findings from the moral distress and moral injury literature.

Moral distress experience in the literature

Jameton makes a distinction between two different types of moral distress: "initial distress" and "reactive distress" (1984). Initial distress is defined as occurring when one first encounters a barrier that prevents a person from acting in the way they believe is moral and is associated with feelings of anger, frustration, and anxiety (McCarthy and Deady, 2008). A blocked MAC represents a "trauma that affects the soul" and violates deeply held moral beliefs, standards, and expectations (Litz et al., 2009; Dombo, Gray, and Earl, 2013). The violation of one's moral schemas produces inner conflict and dissonance where an individual feels a lack of integration of their thoughts, emotions, and understanding of the world (Litz et al., 2009; Vargas et al., 2013; Dombo, Gray, and Earl, 2013). If unresolved, initial moral distress continues and becomes reactive moral distress, which involves complex negative feelings including powerlessness, guilt, and shame (Fry et al., 2002; McCarthy and Deady, 2008; Litz et al., 2009).

While little research discusses the resolution process of moral distress in military HCPs, some research finds that morally distressed service members exhibit a "psychological imperative to reconcile morally incongruent or discrepant experiences" (Litz et al., 2009, p. 701; Fry et al., 2002). Litz and colleagues (2009) describe resolution as involving cognitive and emotional processing as one reflects on a situation and reconstructs more flexible moral schemas that integrates newly learned information, allowing for the healing of moral distress through an "appreciation of context and acceptance of the imperfect self" (p. 703). However, the moral distress resolution process can be experienced either positively or negatively depending on a variety of factors such as one's moral sensitivity, sense of responsibility, and capacity for self-forgiveness (Litz et al., 2009; Bradshaw et al., 2010; Wilkinson, 1987/88).

Findings from both military and civilian HCPs indicate that ongoing reactive and chronically experienced moral distress can lead to progressively more severe consequences. Epstein and Hamric (2009) argue for the incorporation of the related concept of "moral residue" or "that which each of us carries with us from those times in our lives where in the face of moral distress we have seriously compromised ourselves or allowed ourselves to be compromised" (Webster and Baylis, 2000, p. 217). Adding moral residue into the conceptualization of moral distress can account for its progression toward a downward spiral (Epstein and Hamric, 2009). If moral distress is not completely resolved, some moral residue persists, which depletes the individual's baseline for the next encounter with initial moral distress, creating the downward cumulative progression and potential damage from experiencing continuing or chronic moral distress (Epstein and Hamric, 2009; Corley, 2002; Fry et al., 2002; Webster and Baylis, 2000; Wilkinson, 1987/88). Bradshaw and colleagues (2010) find that the residue of unresolved moral distress creates a feedback loop that eventually places an individual in a crisis state, where individuals described a loss of self-control owing to "no longer hav[ing] the resources, both internal and external, to deal with a stressful situation" (p. 72).

Ego-depletion and moral processes

The literature in psychology does not focus on moral distress; however, it offers a useful additional mechanism to consider when discussing cumulative progression of the negative consequences of moral distress. The psychological process of ego-depletion occurs when an individual's limited self-regulation resources that allow them to consciously engage in effortful decision-making and self-control become diminished or exhausted (Baumeister, Gailliot, DeWall, and Oaten, 2006).

Self-regulation

When one encounters challenging and novel situations the application of learned schemas and automatic responses and behaviours may be insufficient when choosing a course of action (Baumeister, Schmeichel, and Vohs, 2007). If so, the self must engage its executive functions to determine how to act: the conscious cognitive processes responsible for deliberating and making effortful choices as well as the regulation of impulses and need gratification (Hagger, Wood, Stiff, and Chatzisarantis, 2010). The executive functions of both self-regulation and self-control "refer to the self's capacity to alter its own states and responses" and are necessary to attain control over one's thoughts, emotions, and behaviours (Baumeister and Mick, 2002; Baumeister, Schmeichel, and Vohs, 2007).

All executive functions are dependent on the consumption of the same pool of "limited resources" that cannot be sustained indefinitely and are akin to the concepts of energy or willpower (Baumeister, Schmeichel, and Vohs, 2007). After efforts involving executive functions, individuals are less effective at successive self-regulatory tasks since these limited resources are vulnerable to deterioration over time from repeated exertions (Hagger et al., 2010). Like a muscle, self-regulation resources can be restored through rest and refraining from self-regulatory tasks as well as through other mechanisms such as meditation (Baumeister, Schmeichel, and Vohs, 2007). If the self is unable to recover these resources, the self enters ego-depletion, a state of diminished resources that must be restored before normal psychological functioning can continue (Baumeister, Gailliot, DeWall and Oaten, 2006; Baumeister, Vohs, and Tice, 2007). Yet, even in an ego-depleted state it is still possible to engage executive functions when the right motivation is in place; however, this continuous depletion of resources produces "severe impairments" in subsequent self-regulation, leading to extensive ego-depletion as well as potentially burnout and other mental health issues (Baumeister, Vohs, and Tice, 2007, p. 353; Rivkin, Diestel, and Schmidt, 2015).

Moreover, resolving self-conscious moral emotions (such as regret, guilt, and shame) necessitates appraisal of the self and external context, which requires use of executive functions, and thus further tax resources and contribute to ego-depletion (Sheikh and Janoff-Bulman, 2010; Harding, 1985). This appraisal involves a self-regulatory feedback loop as the person evaluates the situation, compares it to their moral standards, and attempts to reduce discrepancies between the perceived self and one's standards by self-regulating behaviour (Sheikh and Janoff-Bulman, 2010). The person then again compares the outcome of these adjustments to their moral standards and exits the feedback loop when satisfactory resolution is achieved by either meeting moral standards or altering moral schemas through the integration of new information (Sheikh and Janoff-Bulman, 2010; Dombo, Gray, and Earl, 2013).

Since moral distress requires a self-regulatory feedback loop, which taxes limited resources, it has the potential to lead to ego-depletion as well as difficulty or an inability to resolve and progress through morally distressing situations. If unresolved or encountered chronically, a vicious circle of over-taxing resources creates a cumulative effect that leads to severe ego-depletion and possibly contributes to the development of mental health problems.

Results

EMMRG participants described encountering morally challenging events where their desired choice of action (MAC) was blocked by a barrier (Bradshaw et al., 2010). The barriers consisted of four emerging sorts: (1) lack of resources in the context; (2) the exigencies of the triage system; (3) lack of specialists or specialized knowledge such as where civilian care involved children or palliation; and (4) social and cultural disparities. Contending with a blocked MAC as well as the resulting initial moral distress involved psychological processes that increased self-regulation demands. While resolution processes could help alleviate these demands, the additional stressors of the deployed environment requiring self-regulation created challenges that often thwarted self-reflection. If unresolved, initial moral distress progressed to reactive moral distress that involved additional emotional, psychological, and moral complexities as well as compromised self-regulation. If a participant experienced multiple moral dilemmas that caused moral distress, the consequences were compounded and had cumulative effects on self-regulation.

Encountering a blocked MAC

When first encountering a moral dilemma, the executive function of effortful decision-making is used by individuals who are deliberating on their desired MAC (Sheikh and Janoff-Bulman, 2010). However, when a HCP confronts a barrier to their MAC, they must act in a way contrary to their initial desires. This required participants to suppress or abstain from their MAC and act in another, less desirable way, which involves exercising self-control (Baumeister, Schmeichel, and Vohs, 2007). Participants explained that acting despite a blocked MAC was often painful and led to personal and professional psychological stress. Encountering a moral dilemma that involves a barrier to one's MAC requires that the HCP act in a way that is less ideal and perhaps undesirable, which participants described as requiring self-regulation. EMMRG-22 shared an example of how military HCPs are unable to act in a way they may desire as caregivers because of limitations in the deployed environment. He described his reaction to a situation where he was unable to allocate limited supplies to a patient requiring palliative care because other patients could benefit from the same resources:

> You just feel horrified, you feel, this guy's got a timer on his head counting down as to how much life he has left and you have to tell him "sorry I can't help you." Carry on.
>
> (EMMRG-22)

EMMRG-22 shows the difficulty of being confronted with a barrier to one's desired path in a moral dilemma and the necessity of having to act in a way that is less satisfactory. He explained that acting as a military HCP in a time of scarcity sometimes required him to "carry on" and act in opposition to his initial instincts as a caregiver.

Participants described encountering moral dilemmas that involved a barrier to one's MAC as an experience of psychological difficulty and depletion that often led to professional challenges. EMMRG-11 outlined that her encounters resulted in personal psychological stress and used phrases like "it's hard," "I find that very difficult," and "it's very stressful." EMMRG-07 said her experience with moral distress was one of depletion and exertion: "You are a cross between feeling weak and exhausted." EMMRG-15 explained how barriers to a desired MAC added to the challenges of fulfilling the HCP role: "It's hard for you to be the caregiver ... it's crazy, it's like a constant rollercoaster ride." These difficulties were portrayed by EMMRG-11 as intrinsically painful for military

HCPs, "Yeah, everyone was sort of working in their own little private hell I think." This psychological stress indicates the need for military HCPs to engage the executive functions of self-regulation and effortful decision-making when struggling to act as best as possible, without falling apart, which denotes taxation of the ego's limited resources.

Initial moral distress

Participants' blocked MACs led to emotional upset associated with initial moral distress as well as some compromised abilities to self-regulate emotions and behaviours when reacting to the moral dilemma, suggesting the beginnings of ego-depletion. The negative emotions of anger, frustration, and anxiety were conveyed by participants upon being confronted with a blocked MAC and the resulting initial moral distress. EMMRG participants also described the consequences of initial moral distress as involving intense negative emotions and communicated feelings of disgust and regret for their part in morally distressing events. This indicates that military HCPs identified discrepancies between the actions they felt implicated in and their personal moral standards, inferring the initiation of a self-regulatory feedback loop (Baumeister, Schmeichel, and Vohs, 2007; Sheikh and Janoff-Bulman, 2010).

Participants who had a blocked MAC noted uncharacteristic changes in their ability to exert control over their behaviours and emotions, demonstrating that their ability to self-regulate was compromised when undergoing initial moral distress. EMMRG-01 indicated that she was surprised by her own reaction after a shift in emotional control resulted in a behavioural outburst that she believed was out of character: "I kind of lost it." Another participant described struggling to provide care to an overwhelming number of patients, which resulted in her making an error in patient care that she explained could have been fatal:

> I made a medication error and when I found that out I just stood at the IV pole and I just started to cry {emotional} because it just upset me so much.
>
> (EMMRG-02)

EMMRG-02 showed a diminished capacity to exert self-control over her executive functioning, as indicated by the medication error and atypical over-expression of her emotional reaction. While this compromised self-control may be partly due to the stressors in the deployed work environment; she expressed a connection between experiencing a blocked MAC and an inability to self-regulate her emotions and behaviours. As such, initial moral distress in the deployed environment may lead to self-regulation challenges for military HCPs indicative of the beginnings of ego-depletion (Baumeister, Schmeichel, and Vohs, 2007).

EMMRG participants indicated that acting despite barriers to a desired MAC as well as the resulting initial moral distress contributed to difficulty exercising self-control over their emotional and behavioural reactions. The outcomes of a blocked MAC denoted a need for respondents to practice effortful decision-making and self-regulation, executive functions that tax the ego's limited resources and contribute to depletion. Furthermore, discrepancies between the self and personal moral standards likely begin a self-regulatory feedback loop where the military HCP attempts to meet perceived moral expectations by increasing self-regulation of related behaviours (Baumeister, Schmeichel, and Vohs, 2007; Sheikh and Janoff-Bulman, 2010). Therefore, the initial moral distress at obstruction of intended morally desirable actions engaged the process that could lead to ego-depletion.

Moral distress resolution

While initial moral distress may place demands on the ego's limited resources, engaging in resolution processes could ultimately help to lessen resource demands and ego-depletion by regulating the self's behaviours until moral standards are met or by altering moral schemas to accommodate new information (Dombo, Gray, and Early, 2013; Sheikh and Janoff-Bulman, 2010). Participants outlined attempts to directly address discrepancies between the perceived self and their moral standards by striving to directly alter the situation to remove the barrier blocking their MAC or by moving concerns up the chain of command. Military HCPs also described using self-reflective appraisal to integrate new information into their moral schemas, allowing them to successfully resolve their moral distress:

> Well I just convinced myself that was how it had to be.... I practice medicine exactly as I was trained and I would in Canada until I couldn't and then I didn't and I believe that. So if you can't then it's not your fault anymore.... I don't feel personally responsible ... we made the right decision under the circumstances, but I didn't create the circumstances.... And as a team if we had not been there it would have been much worse, I imagine worse, so we were making things better even if it wasn't 100% solution every time as we would aim for in Canada.
>
> (EMMRG-20)

While EMMRG-20 was sometimes not able to act on her MAC, she explained that she did not feel "personally responsible" because of the influence of uncontrollable contextual elements in the deployed environment. She described engaging in self-reflective appraisal that allowed her to consider and accept those aspects of the moral dilemma that were uncontrollable and then integrated this new information into her moral schemas and expectations regarding personal moral responsibility. However, this appraisal process requires self-control and effortful decision-making, which taxes limited self-regulation resources and may be difficult to achieve depending on the state ego-depletion.

Participants observed that they were often unable to attempt moral distress resolution because of compromised self-regulation associated with challenges in the deployed context, which inherently presents a high frequency of contextual stressors that also require coping and tax self-regulation resources (Gibbons et al., 2013; Owen and Wanzer, 2014; Baumeister, Vohs, and Tice, 2007). (For some, these self-regulation difficulties persisted even after leaving the deployed work environment and negatively affected later resolution processes.) EMMRG-15 described feeling unable to attempt resolution processes due to the pressures of the deployed environment:

> And I always thought to me, to myself I thought you know what, I'm tough I grew up in Toronto, I can get past it. So no matter what comes my way we are just going to work with it and deal with it later. And that was kind of my mentality through the whole thing.
>
> (EMMRG-15)

She adopted a "deal with it later" mentality and avoided attempts at moral distress resolution owing to the additional difficulties of the deployed environment. She explained that while she hoped this mindset would allow her to cope it did not allow for self-reflection, which prevented resolution: "what I was doing was just stuffing it into a closet and not addressing any of it" (EMMRG-15). EMMRG-11 further outlined how the stressors in the environment affected her ability to self-reflect on morally distressing events:

> You're totally in survival mode when you're there, right. The hours are so long the pace is so heavy, the work is so dirty, it's hot, whatever, and you just put your head down and you just do your job. I think it's when you get home and have some time to reflect and to try and sort it all out that ... some of us don't feel very good about what happened
>
> (EMMRG-11)

She described how the stressors inherent in the context were so demanding that she entered "survival mode," which implies difficulty engaging executive functions as they tax self-regulation resources required for coping with deployment and further deplete the ego. Participants portrayed the deployed context as leading to exposure to a heightened number of stressors that made allocating self-regulation resources to moral distress resolution difficult or unfeasible. EMMRG-11 stated that once outside of the demanding deployed environment she felt able to practice self-reflection, but still struggled to fully engage in the resolution processes: "I couldn't even talk about it because it would make me so angry." She explained that she was unable to self-reflect and resolve these challenges because of emotional upset, which signifies compromised self-regulation.

While resolution processes may resolve initial moral distress and lessen ego-depletion by allowing one to exit the self-regulatory feedback loop, many military HCPs found self-reflection difficult owing to already limited resources. Since the resolution process itself consumes self-regulatory resources, the compounded demands on the ego from moral and nonmoral stressors in the deployed context made attempting the resolution of moral distress more challenging. Despite allowing for eventual relief of moral distress, resolution processes engage executive functions that make increasing demands on heavily taxed self-regulation resources and further contribute to ego-depletion. Yet, continuing without resolution when MACs are blocked by contextual forces protracts the self-regulatory feedback loop and advances depletion of the ego.

Reactive moral distress and ego-depletion

When unresolved, initial moral distress persists and becomes reactive moral distress entwined with additional complex emotional and psychological reactions (Jameton, 1984). Reactive moral distress led to participants enduring intense and difficult emotions, such as powerlessness and self-criticism, as well as interruptions to their beliefs and world views. Military HCPs also described experiencing moral emotions when unable to resolve initial moral distress, which are linked with self-regulation demands (Sheikh and Janoff-Bulman, 2010; Gao et al., 2014). Participants described considerable challenges to practicing self-regulation of thoughts, emotions, and behaviours when facing reactive moral distress, indicating significant ego-depletion.

Military HCPs with reactive moral distress described complex negative emotions as well as uncertainty regarding their moral beliefs and roles as military HCPs. Moral emotions such as guilt, shame, and regret also were expressed by participants who were experiencing unresolved reactive moral distress. EMMRG-01 found that she, and other HCPs observed, felt the emotional consequences of reactive moral distress and often blamed themselves for the outcome of a blocked MAC:

> I think there was a lot of internal blame … a lot of us internalize it and are frustrated that we don't know more. I mean we can't know everything about everything.
>
> (EMMRG-01)

Despite acknowledging that overcoming barriers was often not possible, she observed that the tendency of military HCPs was often to internalize self-blame. The resolution of these self-conscious moral emotions necessitates self-reflective appraisal, which places increased demands on self-regulation resources (Sheikh and Janoff-Bulman, 2010).

The consequences of reactive moral distress were associated with significant changes in participants' emotions, thoughts, and behaviours, which demonstrated substantial self-regulation resource depletion in this state. Participants explained that experiences with blocked MACs led to changes regarding their perceived role as military HCP. EMMRG-01 shared how encountering a blocked MAC when struggling to provide care for critically injured children during resource shortages led not only to intense emotions but also to a questioning of her belief systems:

> When children die it just doesn't add up and it just seems too unfair and then you just, people go to a bad place, like what the frig are we even doing here, you know, this is crazy and extremely emotional.
>
> (EMMRG-01)

During reactive moral distress, EMMRG-01 noted that military HCPs "go to a bad place" that leads to the emotional experience of powerlessness, describing how the outcome of a blocked MAC "just doesn't add up" and feeling that the situation is "crazy," implying a perceived lack of control. She told of questioning her role and perceived purpose as a military HCP, indicating uncertainty, self-criticism, and disruption of her moral understanding and beliefs. While this moral disequilibrium and dissonance may be resolved by self-reflection and appraisal, the reconsideration of moral schemas requires executive functions and further taxes self-regulation resources, implying added difficulty when attempting resolution processes (Sheikh and Janoff-Bulman, 2010). EMMRG-22 described frequently being unable to provide sufficient care and resources to an overwhelming number of desperate civilian patients that sometimes inadvertently resulted in conflicts:

> And after a while it gets, if you let it get to you it can get almost demoralizing and make you feel angry and you do not want to help these people.
>
> (EMMRG-22)

EMMRG-22 illustrated that the long-term consequences of unresolved moral distress can impact emotional states as well as thought patterns. He noted an uncharacteristic shift in his perceptions as a military HCP, such that it became difficult to provide care. He attributed this significant change to the "demoralizing" effect of encountering persistent barriers to his desired MAC that went unresolved. This negative shift in his perceptions of his role as a military HCP indicates a compromised ability to self-regulate thoughts and emotions and to maintain normative functioning. Difficulty self-regulating was also expressed by EMMRG-27, who described unresolved moral distress as contributing to challenges performing tasks requiring executive functions:

> I think unresolved issues have a way of spurring you to go back overseas because you feel you have unfinished business. My life kind of came apart a little bit in 2007, I was preparing to go overseas and I realized at the time that one of the reasons I am going or wanted to go overseas so badly was because I had unresolved issues from the first tour. And I needed to prove to myself that I could do this, which is not a good reason to go overseas.
>
> (EMMRG-27)

EMMRG-27 explained that unresolved moral distress was a significant influence and motivation when making his decision to redeploy. He described his desire to "so badly" return overseas as driven by the need to resolve "unfinished business" and prove his ability to function as a military HCP in the deployed environment. He acknowledged that these motivations were not a "good reason" to deploy, but implied that he was unaware of this influence on his decision-making before having a sudden realization as his "life kind of came apart" (EMMRG-27).

For participants, unresolved initial moral distress led to reactive moral distress and was associated with increased difficulty maintaining normative functioning and engaging in executive processes. The accompanying complex moral and nonmoral emotions further taxes self-regulation resources and indicate that a self-regulatory feedback loop is ongoing and not satisfactorily resolved. This contributes to further ego-depletion as demonstrated by participants' compromised abilities to practice decision-making and self-regulation of thoughts, emotions, and behaviours.

Chronic reactive moral distress and extensive ego-depletion

If multiple encounters with morally distressing events occur, as is likely owing to the challenges of working in the deployed context, participants found that the personal outcomes of reactive moral distress were compounded (Litz et al., 2009). Experiencing subsequent morally distressing events was common for EMMRG participants who connected multiple instances of blocked MACs with a cumulative progression of negative psychological consequences. Participants associated this type of "chronic moral distress" with self-regulation failures as well as psychological disorders. Long-term and frequent or "chronic" moral distress was articulated by several EMMRG participants as a risk for military HCPs who were not able to achieve successful resolution. EMMRG-07 described experiencing multiple morally distressing events in her deployment in a conflict zone with high civilian casualties, such as having patients die after being transferred as mandated to local facilities, providing palliative care for severe trauma injuries, and handling bodies being buried in mass graves. The chronic moral distress experienced by EMMRG-07 involved difficulty practicing self-regulation during her deployment which continued after her return:

> The one guy I worked with in [location] my last posting and we were in the platoon together, and we don't talk about it at all, we can't. It's still that raw and it's like, God, it's 18 years ago, you know … and people say "oh you guys were in [location]," conversation over, two people walk in two different directions, it's bad, it's so raw you know.
>
> (EMMRG-07)

She demonstrated difficulty successfully resolving her moral distress, and described continuing to experience negative emotional consequences, even after having been away from the deployed context for 18 years: "it's still that raw." She expressed being completely unable to engage in self-reflection and appraisal of the experience, even with close coworkers from the same team who had similar experiences. She depicted being unable to employ executive functions such as self-regulation in order to attempt appraisal and resolution, describing an inability to discuss the issue and an immediate desire to flee while simultaneously acknowledging that this response was not beneficial: "it's bad." These self-regulation difficulties are indicative of an ongoing feedback loop and severe ego-depletion.

The negative consequences of chronic moral distress were portrayed as increasingly cumulative and resulting in severe consequences for participants such as being unable to redeploy or leaving the profession. After her experiences with chronic unresolved moral distress, EMMRG-07 stated that she lost resilience and was unable to return to the deployed working environment. She shared that her decision to no longer deploy was undesired and disappointing, but necessary to prevent significant personal damage:

> I wasn't able to do it anymore. I kind of think it's like when you're in your early 20s and … you can be hung over or not hung over the next day and then you can go back and do it again on the Saturday night … I don't want to feel like that anymore.… I guess I know the answer but I don't. I just think I have had too many.
>
> (EMMRG-07)

> The reason I got out was because I knew I couldn't deploy anymore and it was difficult {emotional} because it was the thing that I was really good at.… I'm proud of the time I did, but it was a hard pill to swallow.… Because I really think that if I had to deploy again, um, I think I would be done.
>
> (EMMRG-07)

The cumulative effects of unresolved moral distress are demonstrated by EMMRG-07 through the metaphor of alcohol and phrases like "I just think I have had too many" to describe the progression of her experience. Despite feeling proud of her accomplishments as a military HCP, she shared that the compounding consequences prevented her from redeploying, saying decisively that she "couldn't" while indicating that she ideally would have preferred to continue: "it was a tough pill to swallow." This suggests that a self-regulatory feedback loop was unresolved and continued to drain the ego's resources which cumulatively affected her psychological well-being: "at some point you are just really bitter and twisted" (EMMRG-07). She revealed that returning to the deployed context and experiencing additional moral and contextual stress would lead to potentially debilitating negative personal consequences—"I think I would be done"—suggesting a risk of severe ego-depletion leading to significantly compromised normative functioning and mental health concerns.

Other participants directly connected their multiplicity of experiences with unresolved moral distress to the development of stress-related mental health problems, which have been connected to prolonged demands on self-regulation resources (Walter, Gunstad, and Hobfoll, 2010; Rivkin, Diestel, and Schmidt,

2015). Some participants articulated a causative relationship between experiencing barriers in moral dilemmas, being unable to engage in resolution processes, and developing a serious stress disorder. EMMRG-15 described her belief that the development of her PTSD was related to the cumulative effects of long-term psychological demands related to blocked moral challenges:

> in the end, I ended up with PTSD and I also had a lot of issues with some of the ethical things.
>
> (EMMRG-15)

> I don't know if I will ever go back to a theatre of war … when I was diagnosed with PTSD it was because I had long-term chronic stress.
>
> (EMMRG-15)

She explained that, while she felt that she was coping with the consequences effectively ("I thought I was dealing really well" (EMMRG-15)), being continually unable to achieve resolution of her moral distress led to negative psychological health impacts. She stated that during this time she was unstable and did not feel like her normal self, "it took me a year and a half to stabilize it, to start thinking I was normal again" (EMMRG-15). This suggests that unresolved chronic moral distress likely has a cumulative demand on self-regulatory resources owing to the feedback loop and may eventually lead to severe ego-depletion and an inability of the self to maintain stable normal functioning.

EMMRG-01 observed similar difficulties with psychological health in military HCPs, which she attributed to experiencing frequently blocked MACs:

> [Experiencing moral dilemmas] messes up health care professionals and I know many have come back with you know, whether it's PTSD, compassion fatigue, caregiver fatigue, um, vicarious traumatization, whatever, burnout. A lot of it has to do with the ethical dilemmas we are put into.
>
> (EMMRG-01)

She shared her perception that, for many military HCPs, encountering barriers in a moral dilemma and the resulting experience of moral distress are directly related to the development of stress-related psychological health concerns. EMMRG-07 agreed, stating that these consequences could be severe and potentially life-threatening, "[they] were so sick after, you know, and suicidal," depicting how moral distress can be a significant and relentless challenge for many military HCP on deployment.

Discussion

Clear parallels were described by EMMRG participants between the progressive experience of moral distress and the self-regulatory challenges of maintaining normative functioning under conditions of ego-depletion. Military HCP participants depicted their encounters with blocked moral dilemmas as psychologically depleting and involving difficult moral emotions, occurrences that initiate a self-regulatory feedback loop and require engaging executive functions, gradually taxing personal resources. They demonstrated the importance of resolving initial moral distress as well as the difficulty of engaging resolution processes owing to other moral and nonmoral contextual stressors in the deployed environment, which also placed demands on self-regulation resources. If initial moral distress went unresolved, participants described struggling with moral disequilibrium as well as diminished abilities to self-regulate thoughts, emotions, and behaviours; the continuous loop led to ongoing depletion of the ego. When encountering subsequent moral dilemmas involving barriers to their MAC, participants with unresolved moral distress portrayed negative consequences as compounding cumulatively. Military HCPs in this state described heightened difficulty in engaging resolution processes and exhibited significantly compromised abilities to self-regulate indicative of severe ego-depletion, especially if moral distress was experienced chronically. Participants shared their belief that the development of mental health disorders for military HCPs was connected to the experience of chronic moral distress.

This ego-depletion framework based on limited self-regulatory resources may help to further understanding of stress-related mental health challenges facing military HCPs. Military HCPs have been found to develop stress-related psychological illnesses such as compassion fatigue, burnout, depression, and anxiety due to their exposure to medically traumatic experiences rather than combat traumatic experiences (Owen and Wanzer, 2014). Jones and colleagues (2008) found that military HCPs in the UK armed forces were overrepresented in referrals to mental health services, with medical technicians for example composing 3 percent of the armed forces but accounting for 7 percent of psychiatric evacuees. However, little research has examined the consequences of providing morally complex care in the deployed environment on military HCPs' quality of life (Gibbons et al., 2013). While EMMRG participants expressed their belief in a causal link between experiencing moral distress and developing stress-related mental health issues, further research is needed to establish this connection. Since prolonged demands on self-regulatory resources have been associated with stress-related psychological disorders such as PTSD symptoms and burnout, an ego-depletion framework may provide a means of directly connecting morally distressing experiences to the frequently observed negative mental health outcomes for military HCPs (Jones et al., 2008; Walter, Gunstad, and Hobfoll, 2010; Rivkin, Diestel, and Schmidt, 2015). However, more research examining the relationship between ego-depletion and the development of clinical disorders is also essential to verifying this connection and is called for in the psychology literature (Rivkin, Diestel, and Schmidt, 2015; Baumeister, Vohs, and Tice, 2007).

While establishing a correlation between moral distress and mental health would be beneficial for the wellness of individual HCPs, it is also crucial for the effectiveness of the military organization. In civilian HCPs, moral distress is linked with compassion fatigue and burnout; reduced job satisfaction; decreased employee morale; high staff turnover, with 15 percent of nurses having left previous positions owing to moral distress; and lowered retention rates in the department, organization, and profession (Corley, 2002; Davis, Schrader, and Belcheir, 2012; McCarthy and Deady, 2008). As such, any military force concerned about high readiness capability and the ability of HCPs to perform their jobs effectively must be concerned about HCPs' moral well-being, including moral distress (Fry et al., 2002). Understanding the experience of moral distress and its consequences for military HCPs is essential to bolstering individual and team capacities as well as the overall effectiveness of the military organization.

Limitations

There are two potential limiting factors of this chapter: a potential bias when selecting participants, and participants not being asked directly about the concept or experience of "moral distress." First, military HCPs for the EMMRG study were recruited by describing that potential participants would have had experience with "ethical dilemmas"; however, this may have led to more individuals who had experienced an ethical dilemma negatively to participate. If an ethical dilemma had gone unresolved and a person experienced it negatively, the HCP may be more readily able to identify themselves with the study criteria and perhaps even motivated to participate as a means of attempting to address and resolve it. Second, while participants were asked about their experiences with moral dilemmas, the specific terminology of "moral distress" was not explained or used in the interview guide. However, since moral distress by definition is the experience and consequences of encountering a barrier to one's desired MAC in a moral dilemma, it is possible to identify potential moral distress without directly referring to the concept. The experiences of participants who described encountering a barrier to their MAC were included in the analysis.

Conclusion

This analysis suggests evidence for a self-regulatory conceptual basis of moral distress and indicates the potential of a framework based on the psychological mechanism of ego-depletion for understanding the progressive, cumulative experience of moral distress in military HCPs. Encountering a barrier to a MAC and having to act in a way other than desired was stressful and depleting for participants and necessitated resolution processes, all of which involved engaging executive functions. Analysis of participant's narratives also supported the potential applicability of a self-regulatory feedback loop when considering the moral distress resolution process; when military HCPs perceived discrepancies between the self and their moral standards, they exerted self-control over their actions in an attempt to meet their expectations or integrate new information into their moral schemas. Since resolution processes also place demands on limited self-regulation resources, some military HCPs found that the nonmoral and moral stressors compounded and made it difficult to attempt resolution in the deployed environment. As initial moral distress progressed to reactive moral distress, participants described experiencing increased difficulties exerting self-regulation over their thoughts, emotions, and behaviours indicative of progressive ego-depletion (Baumeister, Schmeichel, and Vohs, 2007). The self-regulatory feedback loop involved in ego-depletion also aligns with the effects of moral residue from unresolved moral distress (Epstein and Hamric, 2009), indicating a potential explanation for its cumulative progression and negative consequences for military HCPs, especially when exposure is chronic.

While more practical research is needed to explore and firmly establish these associations, a model that incorporates the mechanism of ego-depletion could potentially advance our knowledge of the moral distress process for HCPs. Connecting moral distress to findings in ego-depletion research provides a theoretical conceptualization of the psychological mechanisms involved at the individual level and may illuminate a possible relationship between the development of moral distress and stress-related mental health issues. If verified, this self-regulatory framework would allow for the extensive findings related to the prevention and recovery of ego-depletion to be applied to the moral distress resolution process, and potentially offer insights into improving care and wellness for morally distressed military HCPs. With a better understanding of the moral distress process and its consequences for individuals and military organizations, we can bolster military HCPs' capacity and willingness to take courageous action in the face of morally challenging situations.

References

Adler, A. B. and Castro, C. A. 2013. An occupational mental health model for the military. *Military Behavioral Health*, 41–51.

Baumeister, R. F., Gailliot, M., DeWall, N. and Oaten, M. 2006. Self-regulation and personality: how interventions increase regulatory success, and how depletion moderates the effects of traits on behavior. *Journal of Personality*, 74(6), 1773–1801.

Baumeister, R. F. and Mick, D. G. 2002. Yielding to temptation: self-control failure, impulsive purchasing, and consumer behavior. *Journal of Consumer Research*, 28(4), 670–676.

Baumeister, R. F., Schmeichel, B. J. and Vohs, K. D. 2007. Self-regulation and the executive function: the self as controlling agent. In A. W. Kruglanski and E. T. Higgins (eds) *Social Psychology: Handbook of Basic Principles*, 2nd edn (pp. 516–539). New York: Guilford.

Baumeister, R. F., Vohs, K. D. and Tice, D. M. 2007. The Strength Model of Self-Control. *Current Directions in Psychological Science*, 16(6), 351–355.

Bradshaw, C. T., Brajtman, S., Cragg, B. and Higuchi, K. 2010. *Canadian Forces Military Nursing Officers and Moral Distress: A Grounded Theory Approach*. Unpublished master's thesis. Ottawa: University of Ottawa.

Corley, M. C. 2002. Nurse moral distress: a proposed theory and research agenda. *Nursing Ethics*, 9(6), 636–650.

Davis, S., Schrader, V. and Belcheir, M. J. 2012. Influencers of ethical beliefs and the impact on moral distress and conscientious objection. *Nursing Ethics*, 738–749.

Dombo, E. A., Gray, C. and Early, B. P. 2013. The trauma of moral injury: beyond the battlefield. *Journal of Religion & Spirituality in Social Work: Social Thought*, 32(3), 197–210.

Epstein, E. G. and Hamric, A. B. 2009. Moral distress, moral residue, and the crescendo effect. *Journal of Clinical Ethics*, 20(4), 330–342.

Fry, S. T., Harvey, R. M., Hurley, A. C. and Foley, B. J. 2002. Development of a model of moral distress in military nursing. *Nursing Ethics*, 9(4), 373–387.

Gao, H., Zhang, Y., Wang, F., Xu, Y., Hong, Y.-Y. and Jiang, J. 2014. Regret causes ego-depletion and finding benefits in the regrettable events alleviates ego-depletion. *The Journal of General Psychology*, 141(3), 169–206.

Gibbons, S. W., Shafer, M., Hickling, E. J. and Ramsey, G. 2013. How do deployed health care providers experience moral injury. *Narative Inquiry in Bioethics*, 3(3), 247–259.

Gustafsson, G., Eriksson, S., Strandberg, G. and Norberg, A. 2010. Burnout and perceptions of conscience among health care personnel: A pilot study. *Nursing Ethics*, 17(1), 23–38.

Hagger, M. S., Wood, C., Stiff, C. and Chatzisarantis, N. 2010. Ego depletion and the strength model of self-control: a meta-analysis. *Psychological Bulletin*, 136(4), 495–525.

Harding, C. 1985. *Moral Dilemmas: Philosophical and Psychological Issues in the Development of Moral Reasoning*. Chicago, IL: Precedent.

Hunt, M. R., Sinding, C. and Schwartz, L. 2012. Tragic choices in humanitarian health work. *Journal of Clinical Ethics*, 23(4), 338–344.

Jameton, A. 1984. *Nursing Practice: The Ethical Issues*. Englewood Cliffs, NJ: Prentice-Hall.

Jones, M., Fear, N. T., Greenberg, N., Jones, N., Hull, L., Hotopf, M., Wessely, S. and Rona, R. J. 2008. Do medical services personnel who deployed to the Iraq war have worse mental health than other deployed personnel? *European Journal of Public Health*, 18(4), 422–427.

Litz, B. T., Stein, N., Delaney, E., Lebowitz, L., Nash, W. P., Silva, C. and Maguen, S. 2009. Moral injury and moral repair in war veterans: A preliminary model and intervention strategy. *Clinical Psychology Review*, 29(8), 695–706.

McCarthy, J. and Deady, R. 2008. Moral distress reconsidered. *Nursing Ethics*, 15(2), 254–262.

Miles, M. B. and Huberman, A. M. 1994. *Qualitative Data Analysis: An Expanded Sourcebook*, 2nd edn. Thousand Oaks, CA: SAGE.

Nilsson, S., Sjöberg, M., Kallenberg, K. and Larsson, G. 2011. Moral stress in international humanitarian aid and rescue operations: a grounded theory study. *Ethics & Behavior*, 21(1), 49–68.

Owen, R. P. and Wanzer, L. 2014. Compassion fatigue in military healthcare teams. *Archives of Psychiatric Nursing*, 28(1), 2–9.

Rivkin, W., Diestel, S. and Schmidt, K.-H. 2015. Psychological detachment: A moderator in the relationship of self-control demands and job strain. *European Journal of Work and Organizational Psychology*, 24(3), 376–388.

Sandelowski, M. 2000. Whatever happened to qualitative description. *Research in Nursing & Health*, 23(4), 334–340.

Schwartz, L., Sinding, C., Hunt, M., Elit, L., Redwood-Campbell, L., Adelson, N., Luther, L., Ranford, J. and DeLaat, S. 2010. Ethics in humanitarian aid word: learning from the narratives of humanitarian health workers. *AJOB Primary Research*, 45–54.

Sheikh, S. and Janoff-Bulman, R. 2010. The "shoulds" and "should nots" of moral emotions: a self-regulatory perspective on shame and guilt. *Personality and Social Psychology Bulletin*, 36(2), 213–224.

Stewart, D. W. 2009. Casualties of war: Compassion fatigue and health care providers. *MEDSURG Nursing*, 18(2), 91–94.

Vargas, A. F., Hanson, T., Kraus, D., Drescher, K. and Foy, D. 2013. Moral injury themes in combat veterans' narrative responses from the National Vietnam Veterans' Readjustment Study. *Traumatology*, 19(3), 243–250.

Walter, K. H., Gunstad, J. and Hobfoll, S. E. 2010. Self-control predicts later symptoms of posttraumatic stress disorder. *Psychological Trauma: Theory, Research, Practice, and Policy*, 2(2), 97–101.

Webster, G. C. and Baylis, F. 2000. Moral residue. In S. B. Rubin and L. Zoloth (eds) *Margin of Error: The Ethics of Mistakes in the Practice of Medicine*. Hagerstown, MD: University Publishing.

Wilkinson, J. M. 1987/88. Moral distress in nursing practice: Experience and effect. *Nursing Forum*, 23(1), 16–29.

Williams-Jones, B., de Laat, S., Hunt, M., Rochon, C., Okhowat, A., Schwartz, L. and Horning, J. 2015. Ethical tensions in the field: the experiences of Canadian military healthcare professionals/Ethische Spannungen im Einsatz—Erfahrungen von kanadischen Militararzten. *Ethics and Armed Forces/Ethik und Militär*, 1, 31–36.

6 Reaching out to Ebola victims

Coercion, persuasion or an appeal for self-sacrifice?[1]

Philippe Calain and Marc Poncin[2]

The Ebola epidemic that devastated three West African countries in 2014–15 will remain a case in point to understand how coercive public health measures can be unsettled and debatable, even in the face of an exceptionally lethal and contagious disease. Furthermore in this emblematic case, ethical considerations about liberty-restricting measures being imposed for the common good of outbreak control were compounded by parallel and acute social or political issues. For example, Sierra Leone and Liberia were just recovering from years of horrific civil wars. Neither had satisfactory legal protections or ethics oversight to be offered when suspected or confirmed cases of Ebola virus disease were compelled to be put in isolation. More universally, it is doubtful if the human rights protections and the ethical conditions that would justify quarantine and isolation could be met in the midst of any major public health disaster.

On the other hand, the West African epidemic triggered a fragmented but massive response from the international community, involving international and humanitarian organizations, the private sector, and aid agencies. Exceptionally, military forces from industrialized countries contributed to this international epidemic response, offering materials, supplies, field hospitals, logistic expertise, and in some case medical personnel to attend Ebola victims. In September 2014, the international president of Médecins Sans Frontières appealed to the United Nations, urging member states to "deploy civilian and military assets" in order to contribute with additional expertise in handling biohazard situations.

Ultimately, the presence of foreign military personnel remained modest in Ebola-affected areas, but it could have created morally problematic situations if the epidemic had kept escalating beyond control. First, foreign military forces engaged in the regional response could have been exposed to the same or additional misperceptions and moral dilemmas as other public health actors, whenever coercive measures were imposed by local authorities. Second, the strict role of military personnel acting as relief providers and health care workers would have been difficult to sustain had the epidemic caused a collapse of national institutions, a breakdown of all public services (including law and order), or a resurgence of civil wars. The thin boundaries between "coercion, persuasion or an appeal for self-sacrifice" are thus particularly relevant to medical military personnel involved in outbreak control.

* * *

Introduction

It is now commonplace to say that the 2014–15 epidemic of Ebola virus disease (EVD) in West Africa has been 'unprecedented', owing to its magnitude, societal impact, regional dimension and international spread. The disarray of local health systems, the mobility of populations, the shortcomings of global health institutions and the absence of an effective regional mechanism for outbreak response are held as prominent reasons for the delayed containment of the epidemic in Guinea, Sierra Leone and Liberia. In such exceptional circumstances, conventional public-health activities to control Ebola outbreaks have magnified unresolved ethical issues and exposed the complexity of tensions between individual autonomy and the common good. Front-line responders striving to implement urgent public-health measures have been working in an unusually difficult context, marked by the temporary suspension of civil liberties, controversial quarantine measures, weak human-rights protection, questionable public-health strategies and blurred responsibilities. These conditions have made encounters between relief workers and Ebola victims ethically problematic and prone to generating moral distress (Ulrich, 2014). This essay will examine how patients' autonomy has been sacrificed to the public-health necessities imposed by the 2014–15 Ebola epidemic. With a focus on forcible isolation, we will develop three problematic dimensions of epidemic-control activities. Firstly, we will argue that socio-political accounts of the frequent resistance of populations to public-health actions have left aside ethical perspectives in general and the question of autonomy in particular. Secondly, we will examine how coercive measures taken during the West African epidemic have failed to meet human rights or ethical standards and how non-governmental actors have reacted to these measures. Thirdly, we will compare the respective strengths of practical and moral reasons that might justify facility isolation with those generally put forward against quarantine. Finally, we will offer recommendations to clarify and ease the position of non-state actors towards coercive measures used in times of major epidemics.

Filovirus outbreaks: explanatory models of resistance and violence

The public-health response to outbreaks of the Ebola and Marburg viruses (members of the *Filoviridae* family, henceforth called 'filovirus') has essentially remained the same since the first verified occurrence of EVD in 1976. For biomedical experts, a number of public-health measures are essential and generally seen as uncontroversial: centralized case isolation (i.e. the management of confirmed cases in designated health-care facilities with maximal biosafety procedures), case finding (through active surveillance, follow-up of rumors and contact tracing), safe burial rites, social mobilization, health promotion and the reinforcement of standard precautions. Other measures remain disputed, for example individual or mass quarantine, border closures or social distancing. Regardless of the scientific authority of public-health prescriptions, collective reactions of fear, disbelief, rumor or hostility have historically been encountered by many relief and scientific teams in their approaches to communities affected by filovirus outbreaks. This was already the case in 1995 when Ebola spread to Kikwit (currently Democratic Republic of the Congo) (Garrett, 2001). In 2001–2002 during an outbreak of EVD in a remote location straddling the border between Gabon and Congo, the reluctance of villagers to collaborate with outbreak-investigation teams created security conditions that forced international members to evacuate the area twice (WHO, 2003). In 2003, health workers received death threats and suffered acts of violence when Ebola broke out again in the same rural setting of Congo (Formenty et al., 2003). Prior to the arrival of researchers, four teachers accused of spreading the disease were assassinated in the town of Kélé. Rural areas are not the only cases. Urban settings have also been the theater of hostility and violence, notably during filovirus outbreaks in Gulu (Uganda) in 2000–2001 (Hewlett and Hewlett, 2005) and in Uige (Angola) in 2005 (Roddy et al., 2007).

Unsurprisingly West Africa has experienced the same sort of reactions, whereby national and international teams tasked with public-health activities have been facing recurrent and widespread hostility from many affected communities. There are frequent reports of patients in hiding or refusing to present to treatment facilities. In Sierra Leone, during the most recent period of enforced lockdown, systematic home searches found that about one third of all patients had previously not been identified by contact tracing (Sahid, 2015). In Guinea, the frequency of incidents has been monitored by Guinean authorities since November, 2014 (Reliefweb, 2015) by recording the weekly number of sub-prefectures reporting *réticences*. *Réticences* (as opposed to the more politically charged "resistance") is a neutral qualifier that encompasses all instances of opposition to either contact tracing, transfer to isolation, safe burials or other public-health interventions (ACAPS, 2015a). Examples given in national weekly reports include the refusal to be put in isolation, verbal violence, vandalism, death threats, the stoning of cars or physical aggression towards outreach teams. In Guinea, the geographical spread of *réticences* culminated in January, 2015, with 32 of the 341 sub-prefectures or urban communes reporting incidents. As of April, 2015 a few areas close to the capital city of Conakry remained hostile to outreach teams. Local measures taken by the Guinean authorities have generally focused on mass communication and interventions by peers, religious leaders or traditional authorities. In January 2015, the President of Guinea authorized the use of force against those who oppose to Ebola control measures (Diallo, 2015). The open epidemiological category of *réticences* is misleading, as it conflates two morally distinct actions, i.e. the legitimate reluctance of individuals to comply with extreme public-health measures and genuine acts of violence. On top of minor daily incidents, a number of extremely violent events have affected and delayed the work of relief organizations. On 4 April, 2014 in Guinea, less than three weeks after the confirmation of the outbreak, mobs in the town of Macenta threatened Médecins Sans Frontières (MSF) teams, forcing the suspension of all Ebola-control activities for one week. In September 2014 in Womey (Forest region, Guinea) eight members of a high-ranking delegation were murdered, including three health officials. The same month, Red Cross teams collecting dead bodies were attacked in the mining town of Forecariah. In Sierra Leone, similar incidents occurred in Koidu in October, 2014, leaving two dead and residents under curfew (Ruble, 2014). The incident followed an attempt by health officials, to take an elderly woman to an Ebola treatment center against the will of family members. In Liberia, the township of West Point in Monrovia was the theater of major incidents in August 2014 after mobs looted an Ebola clinic. Soon after, clashes with security forces followed quarantine and curfew orders, leaving many wounded and one dead from gunshot wounds.

The political dimension of civil unrest that accompanies major Ebola outbreaks is omnipresent and complex. In West Africa, opposition to public health authorities has been interpreted as an expression of the social divisions left successively by the colonization, civil wars, and post-conflict development policies. In Guinea for example, the frequent resistance to Ebola-response activities reflects both historical and contemporary factors, themselves influenced by national and international circumstances. In the Forest region, where the Ebola epidemic started, long-lasting secular conflicts still divide communities and generate mistrust against national authorities (Anoko, 2015). In addition, memories of coercive public health measures during the colonial era, mixed with resentment about past international clinical trials entertain rumors of an intentional origin of the disease (ACAPS, 2015b). Putting the epidemic in a broader international context, Wilkinson and Leach (2015) see local resistances to epidemic response as a consequence of the structural violence and inequalities that prevail in post-colonial Africa, exacerbated by the inevitable presence of foreign or international agencies working in support of national authorities. Examining international biomedical perspectives, Leach and Hewlett (2010) have shown how a 'global outbreak' narrative pervades health policies and their interpretation of epidemic events. This narrative privileges scientific authority over local knowledge and calls for external remediation, ignoring how popular knowledge can integrate with biomedical science. In a narrow interpretation, the global outbreak narrative shifts the blame to victims, variably accused of medical superstitions, unsafe burials, consumption of infectious wild game, or the shunning of Ebola treatment centers.

Aside from political contexts, medical anthropology provides another explanatory framework. With their pioneering field work in Uganda (Hewlett and Hewlett, 2008), Congo (Formenty et al., 2003; Hewlett et al., 2005) and Gabon (Hewlett and Hewlett, 2008), anthropologists have documented how hostile reactions to public-health measures reflect a divide between biomedical representations of EVD and other cultural models prevailing in African societies. For example, traditional and biomedical communities would typically diverge in their interpretations of disease, contagion and healing, in the way they conduct protective rituals, in their handling of the deceased during burial rites, or in their understanding of risk groups and sources of the disease. Anthropological approaches are essential to guide the response to filovirus epidemics through community engagement (Epelboin, 2015; Marais et al., 2016), mediation (Anoko, 2015) and flexibility in the application of biomedical models (Chandler et al., 2015). At the same time, anthropological perspectives are incomplete and run the risk of patronizing interpretations if cultural aspects of resistances are taken at face value. Cultural explanations alone discount the capacity for autonomous decision-making, expected from anyone exposed to the consequences of contagion and regardless of national or cultural affiliations. In other words, reactions of disbelief or opposition to public-health measures are rational and universal and would likely be felt by many of us facing the prospect of quarantine, isolation, social ostracism, suffering and possible death. Practically, communities are keen to incorporate traditional and biomedical models in a form of medical pluralism compatible with epidemic control protocols (Hewlett and Amola, 2003). Recent work establishes how rural or urban communities can naturally adjust public health necessities to their material and social constraints. For example, Richards et al. (2015) describe the rural settlement of Fogbo in Sierra Leone, and the complexity of social factors of transmission of EVD in a community sustaining itself through family help, kinship, migration, and local markets. In Liberia, Abramowitz et al. (2015) analyse how urban communities managed to organise themselves to contain the outbreak, when left on their own without outside assistance. Thus, local knowledge can bring about efficient survival strategies, particularly when the state and international response are failing. When liberty-restricting measures are imposed in this context, they are bound to exacerbate pre-existing tensions, whereas trustworthiness and reciprocity should be put forward instead. Trust in local institutions (Richards et al., 2015) and hospitals (Brown and Kelly, 2014) are important for communities to seek help for EVD. Focus-group discussions conducted in Monrovia in November, 2014 (Kutalek et al., 2015) revealed additional concerns. Local participants rejected an incentive scheme intended to increase the reporting of suspected cases and pointed out specific problems compromising the credibility of public-health actions, e.g. food shortages for families in quarantine, communication between patients and their families, basic health services, psychosocial support for affected families and the inclusion of Ebola survivors in the teams of active casefinders and contact-tracers.

Quarantine and restrictions of freedom

Around July–August, 2014, four countries (Guinea, Liberia, Nigeria and Sierra Leone) in an attempt to contain the Ebola epidemic issued emergency presidential declarations and a comprehensive list of compulsory measures. The range of legal prescriptions varied from country to country, drawing from the following categories of measures: closures of public places, compulsory leave, *cordon sanitaire*, curfews, sanitation, isolation, price control, quarantine, screening, surveillance, testing, travel restrictions and treatment (Hodge et al., 2014). Mali and Senegal—other African countries that faced the threat of Ebola propagation—also resorted to active surveillance, quarantine and isolation.

At the very least, coercive public-health measures need to be based on compelling scientific evidence and framed in clear and consistent legal and ethical principles (Rothstein, 2015a). The following analysis shows that this does not seem to have been the case during Ebola epidemics, particularly in West Africa. Quarantine has so far been the most disputed issue among other public-health measures prescribed and enforced by public authorities. In contrast, isolation has usually been granted as an absolute necessity in the face of acute epidemics of highly lethal communicable diseases, and it has therefore been seen as ethically unproblematic. For example, commenting on the SARS epidemic, Wynia (2007) claimed that the isolation of sick patients 'tends not to provoke much concern', compared to the quarantine of healthy people. To the contrary, we contend that the isolation of EVD patients raises different but not less concerning questions than other liberty-restricting measures.

Human rights law

The remit of liberty-restricting measures in response to public-health emergencies can be analyzed from at least three different angles, i.e. national laws, the human rights doctrine (embodied in International Human Rights Law) and ethics. The enforcement of laws and treaties, including International Human Rights Law (IHRL), is the responsibility of States. As an element of IHRL, the UN Siracusa Principles (United Nations, 1985) spell out criteria for suspending civil and political rights in case of public emergencies. These include threats to public-health, as specified in Article 25:

> Public health may be invoked as a ground for limiting certain rights in order to allow a state to take measures dealing with a serious threat to the health of the population or individual members of the population. These measures must be specifically aimed at preventing disease or injury or providing care for the sick and injured.

According to the Siracusa principles, restrictions to civil liberties should meet the criteria of being (i) provided for and carried out in accordance with the law, (ii) in the interests of a legitimate objective of general good, (iii) strictly necessary in a democratic society to achieve the objective, (iv) the least intrusive and restrictive means available to reach the same objective, (v) based on scientific evidence, and (vi) not imposed arbitrarily or in a discriminatory manner (WHO, 2007). Furthermore, exceptional measures should be of limited duration and subject to review and appeal (Rothstein et al., 2003). In this context it is important to specify the roles and responsibilities of international and non-governmental organizations. Non-governmental agencies that simultaneously provide the expertise, materials and extra human capacity needed to contain an epidemic are inevitably at risk of misperceptions about their role in the implementation of restrictive measures. This could ostensibly be the case, for example, when protection by the police is sought to reach victims or when security forces themselves need training in or protection from biohazards. Regardless of the relevance of coercive measures imposed by national states of emergency, non-governmental medical agencies have no role or legitimacy in enforcing public-health measures. They are bound to respect national laws, but they cannot possibly be held accountable for the enforcement of public-health law. Neither international humanitarian law nor common ethical principles would justify such powers. In addition, the fact that none of the emergency public health laws have been declared by way of proclamation (Karimova, 2015) by West African countries could invalidate the derogations to the International Covenant on Civil and Political Rights that they represent.

Ethical pragmatism

While lacking the force of law, public-health ethics recognize the necessity that some collective actions should outweigh individual autonomy. Ethicists (Presidential Commission for the Study of Bioethical Issues, 2015; Rothstein, 2015b) have reached very similar conclusions to the Siracusa principles, by enunciating ethical principles governing quarantine and other restrictive measures during public-health emergencies. These ethical principles can be summarized as public necessity, demonstrated effectiveness and scientific rationale, proportionality and least infringement, reciprocity, justice and fairness. The same or similar principles derive from several public health ethics frameworks, indicating on what conditions the common good could outweigh individual autonomy in case of public health necessity (reviewed in Bensimon and Upshur, 2007). As recent epidemic crises have shown (HIV/AIDS, multidrug-resistant tuberculosis, SARS and pandemic influenza), coercive measures are highly contextual and always controversial. The Ebola crisis has precisely exposed the limits of established ethics frameworks, in their contextual and pragmatic applications. Ethical principles have remained at best distant declarations of intent, and ethics debates have largely been sidestepped in programmatic decisions. Reflecting on quarantine and isolation from different perspectives, the following considerations lead to the very concrete point of ethical tension, where the persuasions of public health meet individual autonomy.

Compelling evidence?

With their rapid developments, influenza pandemics (MacPhail, 2014) and the SARS epidemic of 2003 are cases in point for contemporary debates about quarantine. In the case of SARS, the effectiveness of quarantine—compared to isolation alone—is still debated (Day et al., 2006; Barbisch et al., 2015), and the strength of available scientific evidence depends on variable methodological or statistical assumptions (Bondy et al., 2009). Ethicists (Bensimon and Upshur, 2007) have emphasized the contingent nature of scientific evidence and the inherent risk of deriving hasty or definitive decisions about quarantine from limited scientific information. Semantic precision is also important. At first glance, definitions are clear (Presidential Commission for the Study of Bioethical Issues, 2015). Quarantine is the "separation of persons exposed to but not exhibiting symptoms of a communicable disease". Isolation is the "separation of those infected with or exhibiting symptoms of a communicable disease". Still, we are left to define (i) what "separation" means practically, (ii) what kind of symptoms count, and (iii) what type of exposure counts. Furthermore, separation can be forcible or voluntary and entail varying degrees of social distancing. Persons infected with SARS or influenza shed viruses before becoming symptomatic. This is unlike the case of EVD, where persons infected with current filovirus strains are not contagious until they display symptoms of the illness (Racaniello, 2014). The difference is important for both practical and moral reasons. The quarantine of asymptomatic SARS and influenza contacts could plausibly limit the odds of silent transmission in a community. In the sense of being non-discriminatory, it is a genuine public-health measure. The quarantine of asymptomatic Ebola contacts does not fulfill the same epidemiological rationale. Instead of primarily limiting viral spread, Ebola quarantine is a measure to control the movement of people deemed untrustworthy for reporting their symptoms. It is therefore more open to discrimination and arbitrary enforcement.

It is simply plausible that the voluntary or compulsory quarantine of household contacts may play a role in the rapid containment of filovirus outbreaks detected at their very early stage. In Nigeria (Grigg et al., 2015) and Mali (Diallo and Felix, 2014), index cases could be identified rapidly in urban settings, and quarantine measures were applied to all traceable contacts. In Nigeria group quarantine was also imposed upon a minority of contacts posing particular risks of further transmission due to their occupations or home environments. As for mass quarantine (*cordon sanitaire*), it was probably ineffective in Kikwit in 1995 (Heymann, 2014), although this claim has also been questioned (Garrett, 2014).

Quarantine here and abroad

For persons exposed to Ebola, the 2014 interim US guidance (Centers for Disease Control and Prevention, 2014) provided some clarity by distinguishing between "active and direct monitoring", "controlled movement", "exclusion from public places" and "exclusion from the workplace". The same document gives clear definitions of risk categories, clinical criteria and derived public-health actions. It addresses the case of individual persons exposed to Ebola but remains silent about collective or mass actions.

Forcible quarantine measures implemented in West African countries are qualitatively different from public-health actions considered in the US public-health guidance. They fall in a normative vacuum of international guidance and certainly lack compelling scientific evidence. Significantly, in West Africa the forcible quarantine of entire Ebola-exposed families or communities has dramatic consequences. Their stigmatization is one aspect. Furthermore, the temporary loss of livelihoods and basic commodities makes quarantine practically unsustainable for poor families already taxed by the loss of relatives (Kutalek et al., 2015; ACAPS, 2015a). The distribution of food supplies to quarantined households has remained a marginal solution (ACAPS, 2015a). Anecdotal evidence (Bianchi, 2015) indicates that some patients admitted to isolation wards conceal their exact address as a way to protect their families from the dire consequences of quarantine.

Issued at the end of July, 2014, the West African emergency declarations did not cause much international outcry. It is troubling that forcible quarantine and isolation started to elicit reactions in Western countries only late in October, 2014, when expatriate workers returning to the US became themselves subject to liberty-restricting measures imposed by their own state jurisdictions. In the USA, the much publicized case of Ms. Kaci Hickox, a MSF volunteer returning from Sierra Leone, unfolded successively as episodes of forcible isolation, home quarantine and controlled displacements (Miles, 2015). The controversy had multiple dimensions, i.e. human rights issues, the relevance of imposed restrictions from a public-health perspective, doubts about the existence of symptoms, inconsistencies between US federal, state or military prescriptions and the relative discomfort of being detained in makeshift conditions of isolation. As a trained MSF Ebola nurse, Ms. Hickox denied any unprotected exposure to the virus and objected to any restriction of movement which put her at odds with state authorities. In support to her views, scholars (Drazen et al., 2014; Koenig, 2015) and others (MSF, 2014) have put forward a number of arguments against the forcible quarantine of healthy volunteers returning from epidemic-hit countries, e.g. the fragmentation of public-health agencies, the inconsistencies of public-health laws between states, practical obstacles to the implementation of coercive measures, solidarity with and respect of aid workers, evidence that active monitoring and voluntary distancing are sufficient public-health measures and deterring the enrollment of other volunteer workers because of unnecessarily restrictive measures.

Thus legal, ethical and pragmatic reasons for rejecting EVD quarantine are partly different for West Africa and industrialized countries. Regardless, it would be inconsistent for international organizations to oppose quarantine orders in the USA while at the same time remaining silent on forcible quarantine in West Africa. Except perhaps for the early stages of Ebola epidemics, it appears that collective and forcible quarantine actions have failed on the grounds of public necessity, demonstrated effectiveness and scientific rationale. Concerning proportionality, least infringement, reciprocity, due process and the ability to lodge legal appeals, quarantine for EVD does not meet ethical and human-rights standards either in a context of national disaster and weak institutions.

Facility isolation: an onerous public-health measure

So far we have examined the shortcomings of the compulsory quarantine of EVD-patient contacts. Likewise, it is legitimate to next ask how the isolation of symptomatic patients meets the conditions imposed by international human-right law and ethics, including compelling scientific evidence. Two related questions await empirical research with survivors or the families of victims. To what extent does facility isolation reflect free choice, persuasion or some sort of coercion imposed by emergency circumstances or by the absence of any alternative option? What proportion of individuals would be ready to sacrifice themselves for the sake of the common good by entering isolation units for the sole reason of protecting their households and communities from contagion? These two questions can be approached together by preliminary considerations about the current rationale for isolation and its consequences.

The meaning of isolation

There is historical and theoretical evidence that the isolation of cases is one of the most essential measures to contain EVD (Pandey et al., 2014), together with safe burial practices and contact tracing. Yet the consequences of isolation are often shrouded by emergency considerations. Even more than with quarantine, individuals subjected to facility isolation experience extraordinary limitations to their autonomy, particularly in the circumstances of mass catastrophes. Their distress is aggravated by a sudden and sometimes definitive separation from relatives or by the frequent destruction of their few belongings for disinfection. Once in isolation, patients are allegedly free to leave, although the "escape" of patients has occasionally created difficult situations, to which relief teams have felt obliged to react forcefully (Fink, 2015). More recently in Sierra Leone, "escapees" have been publicly named and shamed by national authorities (Mac Johnson and Larson, 2015). In typical Ebola management facilities (also called Ebola Treatment Centers or Units) isolation has at least four dimensions: physical, cognitive, affective and spiritual. To avoid any risk of physical contact with patients' bodies or fluids, mainstream standards of protective equipment call for full body coverage for attending professionals. As a consequence, cultural or linguistic barriers are compounded by additional obstacles to verbal and facial communication and by the rapid rotation of care takers exposed to hyperthermia (Sprecher et al., 2015). With these conditions, patients are inevitably left in a degree of cognitive isolation by being limited in their capacity to know about their condition, their prognosis and the state of their families. As the epidemic became more manageable in West Africa, MSF and other organizations have introduced architectural adjustments to facilitate contact between patients in isolation and relatives, survivors or even religious leaders. Unfortunately, cognitive, affective and spiritual isolation remain difficult to alleviate for the most incapacitated cases, particularly when they are close to death. A most distressing situation experienced by health personnel has been the isolation of children, many of whom have been orphaned by their parents' death from EVD (Zellmann, 2015; Maron, 2015). Contrary to earlier practices, current isolation protocols fail to account for different degrees of exposure in isolation zones, making the presence of relatives at the bedside generally impossible.

Isolation paradigms

The model of isolation in centralized facilities equipped with maximal biosecurity has become a norm for pragmatic and staffing reasons. From a pure public-health perspective, there is no doubt that facility isolation in 'treatment beds' had a major impact on the reduction of disease transmission in West Africa (Kucharski et al. 2015a). This is not to say that it has always been an absolute necessity, in particular where the social cost could have outweighed direct public health gains. Based on the epidemic parameters of 2014, projections (Merler et al., 2015) suggest that epidemic control could be achieved, together with other critical measures, when 70% of the cases become isolated either in Ebola treatment units, at home or in community settings. Smaller community care centers (CCCs) would increase the acceptance of isolation. In theory, in terms of epidemic control CCCs could be as effective as Ebola treatment units (Witty et al., 2014; Washington and Meltzer, 2015), but they require equally strict infection-control procedures (Kucharski et al., 2015b).

Home-based isolation was used in previous filovirus epidemics to offer alternative options to those unwilling to be hospitalized (Kerstiëns and Matthys, 1999; Formenty et al., 2003; Roddy et al., 2007). For example, MSF has guidelines for "home-based support and risk reduction", a procedure where a single caregiver is allowed to provide minimal care after receiving training, protective equipment and sanitary supplies (Sterk, 2008). A review of epidemiological observations in past filovirus outbreaks indicates that family attendants sharing a room with patients are at much lower risk of contamination if they are not involved in direct nursing care (Shears and O'Dempsey, 2015). One can thus assume that minimal care (e.g. handling food and drink) can safely be offered at home under reduced protective clothing and after appropriate training of designated attendants. Thus, depending on the circumstances or phases of an EVD outbreak, facility isolation does not necessarily represent the only option or is the least intrusive and restrictive means available. While we are still unsure about how much risk-reduction other models might afford, the pragmatic limits of centralized facility isolation were reached in the summer of 2014 during the peak of urban transmission of Ebola in Monrovia. When response teams became overwhelmed, clear criteria for prioritizing access to facility admissions were inexistent, and urban communities were ready to become self-reliant in managing essential outbreak-control activities (Abramowitz et al., 2015).

For EVD patients, facility isolation thus represents the most onerous among currently prescribed public-health measures. It is therefore not surprising that the prospect of forcible isolation has contributed to fears and hostility from many Ebola victims towards outreach teams.

Reaching out to Ebola patients: an ethical quagmire

Implicit and explicit reasons for isolation

Obviously from a medical perspective, the fact that case-isolation is imposed by law does not imply that the patients' autonomy should be disregarded. Unless outreach teams represent public-health or law-enforcement authorities, the use of overt coercion would be illegal and in any case ethically problematic for health professionals. This is even more so for foreign humanitarian workers, who have neither the legal authority nor an international mandate to enforce public-health measures. It is also doubtful whether patients would have the possibility of legal recourse to oppose isolation orders in the event of a major Ebola epidemic outbreak in Western Africa. Leaving aside the legality and relevance of coercive measures, let us now assume for a moment that isolation is largely voluntary with patients either presenting spontaneously at the gates of treatment units or being willingly transferred from home after being notified they were a suspected case. To respect patients' dignity, their choices need to be informed by genuine reasons for isolation. These reasons are not always made explicit, consistent or clear by the health community.

As discussed earlier, a first and prominent reason to follow measures of isolation is to *limit contagion* and offer the material possibilities of being cared for at a safe distance from unprotected relatives. While the argument is compelling from a public-health perspective, patients are ultimately asked to sacrifice themselves for the common good or the safety of their families.

A less altruistic but a more convincing reason to enter isolation would be to *receive better care* and to improve one's chances of survival. This argument has been increasingly emphasized in health-promotion messages. In reality there is little evidence in claiming that the current clinical management in dedicated isolation units consistently and significantly guarantees better chances of survival in Africa. Intensive care guided by basic monitoring of biological parameters certainly makes a difference in terms of survival (Lyon et al., 2014), but local capacities for such care are still inconsistent and sparse. However deplorable, this reality should be disclosed without ambiguity to all persons advised to seek care in isolation facilities. One could argue that the combined conditions of emergency and unrest would justify some degree of deception to achieve overarching public-health goals and public safety. Such a position would be in any case ethically problematic—and even more questionable in the future—with the increasing availability of experimental interventions. The latter will introduce the added dimension of consent to research in this difficult context and make the obligation of veracity toward patients and communities the more pressing. Telling the truth about limited treatment capacities does not mean relinquishing hope. In this regard, the role of survivors as witnesses and trusted sources of information about the reality of isolation (USAID, 2015) is fundamental.

Aside from better clinical care and reduced transmission, there are still other reasons for patients to opt for facility isolation, for example the *pressure applied by an unsupportive or hostile community*. Infrequently, the *mental capacity* of patients could be affected by the disease. This would be an exceptionally difficult situation, if it put attendants and medical personnel at increased risk. It would however be inappropriate to assume that most Ebola patients suffer from impaired cognition, even at an advanced stage of the disease. Instead, they should primarily be seen as autonomous persons, capable of choice, but placed in a position of vulnerability by the severity of the disease, the circumstances and, sometimes, by the intimidating deployment of protective paraphernalia.

Ethics principles translated in action

We now come back to the critical and ethically problematic encounter, which is central to this paper. Contact tracers and case finders have testified on how they often found themselves facing moral dilemmas, when public-health actions to limit contagion conflicted with their obligation to respect patients' autonomy and dignity. What remained available to them was the force of persuasion and appeals to self-sacrifice, making it difficult to find the appropriate balance between persuasion and subtle coercion, or between veracity and deception. From what precedes, and combining ethical principles with pragmatic observations, we propose six practical recommendations for medical outreach teams to avoid the pitfalls of coercion when approaching suspected EVD cases (Box 6.1). These recommendations all express moral deference for individual autonomy and dignity, while specific recommendations translate obligations of trustworthiness, reciprocity, and proportionality. These moral obligations seem to us the most essential ones, as they connect with the expectations of affected communities. They are likely to reinforce trust and ease tensions, and they would

---

Box 6.1 Practical ethical guidance to outreach teams

Trustworthiness

- Veracity: openness about the exact reasons—with their burdens and benefits—for isolation
- Clarity of roles: separation from law enforcement authorities
- The inclusion of Ebola survivors in outreach teams

Reciprocity

- Material and psychological support for families
- The provision of basic health services

Proportionality and least infringement

- The offering of genuine choices: possible alternatives to facility isolation, including home-based care

---

probably contribute to reducing community transmission by overcoming hostility, miscommunication and the hiding of victims (Meltzer et al., 2014). While veracity and clarity of roles are unconditional, other actions are progressively achievable, depending on the context. For example, the acute phase of the disaster-response might initially justify inflexible procedures with little space for such considerations as the provision of basic health services or the follow-up of some Ebola patients at home. Offering all possible choices, including alternatives to facility isolation might represent a trade-off between infection control and autonomy. We believe that this trade-off is ethically sound, and practically manageable through sensible processes of community involvement. In any case, the conduct of therapeutic trials in treatment centers cannot be ethically defensible as long as patients have not freely consented to facility isolation.

Conclusions

During the West African Ebola epidemic, the practical limits of upholding human rights and ethical principles have been put to the test for medical teams tasked with the application of public-health measures. Perhaps more than others, members of outreach teams have faced practical and moral issues when tasked with identifying cases in communities and transporting them to centralized isolation facilities. This is not only due to the constant threat of contamination but also to the concurrent circumstances imposed by (i) states of emergency accompanied by forcible public-health prescriptions and (ii) the frequently encountered hostility of affected communities.

In this essay we have discussed how both quarantine and isolation enforced in West Africa after declarations of states of emergency became equally problematic in the light of human rights and ethical perspectives. They deserve the same public scrutiny as the isolated cases of coercion seen in industrialized countries with home-coming humanitarian professionals. Forceful quarantine has probably contributed little to curbing the epidemic. On the other hand, facility isolation has been imposed by a clearer public-health rationale but also at some moral cost and in the absence of consistent ethical guidance. We are unsure if facility isolation was an absolute and constant necessity in the course of the epidemic. The prospect of being kept in isolation may at times have created deterrence in communities and contributed to the perpetuation of the epidemic. We would thus propose a series of pragmatic recommendations aimed at easing tensions between relief workers and communities while respecting the autonomy of the victims of epidemic disasters. We recognize that some of these recommendations are progressively achievable, depending on the specific stage or setting of an outbreak. At the same time, as circumstances evolve, respect for patients' choices should prevail. With the prospect of new therapeutic or preventive interventions, new designs of containment techniques or parallel actions to support health systems, the response to filovirus outbreaks might be different in the future. Still, complex ethical challenges will inevitably be encountered when the context imposes the co-existence of disputed public-health actions, coercive laws and the carrying out of research. Disastrous circumstances can happen with any public health event of national or international concern. Our recommendations are therefore generic, beyond the specific case of filovirus epidemics.

According to a dominant worldview, the West African situation is a regional exception explained by political and socio-cultural circumstances, dysfunctional health systems and weak public institutions. We to the contrary see it more as an exemplary and universal case, anticipating what would happen when epidemic disasters impose measures that are unpopular and onerous to civil liberties and communal values. Taken alone, political or socio-cultural explanations tend to play down the autonomy of affected individuals and reduce their lack of compliance with public-health measures to an African singularity. An ethics analysis opens broader perspectives, recognizing the importance of autonomy and the failure of authoritarian approaches to outbreak control.

Notes

1 This chapter was first published under the same title in *Social Science & Medicine*, 17 (2015), 126–133. Copyright Elsevier. Reprinted with permission.

The main ideas of this chapter were presented and discussed by the first author at the Fifth ICMM Workshop on Military Medical Ethics held in Ermatingen (Switzerland) in May 2015. The paragraphs before the Introduction were added for this reprint.

2 The authors thank the following colleagues for thoughtful reviews of an earlier draft of this manuscript: Caroline Abu Sa'Da, Sergio Bianchi, Iza Ciglenecki, Fernanda Falero, Satoru Ida, Anja Wolz. We are also grateful to Mireille Lador for systematic searches of press archives, and to Timothy Fox for proofreading this version.

References

Abramowitz, S. A., McLean, K. E., McKune, S. L., Bardosh, K. L., Fallah, M., Monger, J., Tehoungue, K. and Omidian, P. A. 2015. Community-centered responses to ebola in urban Liberia: the view from below. *PLoS Negl Trop Dis* 9(4): e0003706. Available online at www.ncbi.nlm.nih.gov/pmc/articles/PMC4391876/

ACAPS. 2015a. *Ebola Outbreak in West Africa. Lessons Learned from Quarantine – Sierra Leone and Liberia.* 19 March 2015. Available online at http://acaps.org/img/documents/t-acaps_thematic_note_ebola_west_africa_quarantine_sierra_leone_liberia_19_march_2015.pdf.

ACAPS. 2015b. *Ebola in West Africa. Guinea: Resistance to the Ebola Response.* 24 April 2015. Available online at http://acaps.org/img/documents/t-acaps_ebola_guinea-resistance-to-ebola-response_24-april-2015.pdf.

Anoko, J. 2015. *Communication with Rebellious Communities during an Outbreak of Ebola Virus Disease in Guinea: An Anthropological Approach.* Ebola Response Anthropology Platform. Available online at www.ebola-anthropology.net/case_studies/communication-with-rebellious-communities-during-an-outbreak-of-ebola-virus-disease-in-guinea-an-anthropological-approach.

Barbisch, D., Koenig, K. L. and Shih, F. Y. 2015. Is there a case for quarantine? Perspectives from SARS to Ebola. *Disaster Medicine and Public Health Preparedness*, 9(5), 547–553.

Bensimon, C. M. and Upshur, R. E. G. 2007. Evidence and effectiveness for decision making for quarantine. *American Journal of Public Health*, 97(suppl 1), S44–S48.

Available online at www.ncbi.nlm.nih.gov/pmc/articles/PMC1854977/pdf/0970044.pdf.

Bianchi, S. 2015. *Determinants of Ebola Health Seeking Behaviors: Reflections from Freetown, Sierra Leone, MSF-UREPH*. Internal report, May 2015.

Bondy, S. J., Russell, M. L., Laflèche, J. M. and Rea, E. 2009. Quantifying the impact of community quarantine on SARS transmission in Ontario: estimation of secondary case count difference and number needed to quarantine. *BMC Public Health*, 9, 488. Available online at www.ncbi.nlm.nih.gov/pmc/articles/PMC2808319.

Brown, H. and Kelly, A. H. 2014. Material proximities and hotspots: toward an anthropology of viral hemorrhagic fevers. *Medical Anthropology* Quarterly, 28(2), 280–303. Available online at www.ncbi.nlm.nih.gov/pmc/articles/PMC4305216/pdf/maq0028-0280.pdf.

Centers for Disease Control and Prevention. 2014. *Interim U.S. Guidance for Monitoring and Movement of Persons with Potential Ebola Virus Exposure*. 24 December 2014. Available online at www.cdc.gov/vhf/ebola/exposure/monitoring-and-movement-of-persons-with-exposure.html.

Chandler, C., Fairhead, J., Kelly, A., Leach, M., Martineau, F., Mokuwa, E., Parker, M., Richards, P. and Wilkinson, A. 2015. Ebola: limitations of correcting misinformation. *Lancet*, 385, 1275–1277. Available online at www.thelancet.com/journals/lancet/article/PIIS0140-6736%2814%2962382-5/fulltext?rss=yes.

Day, T., Park, A., Madras, N., Gumel, A. and Wu, J. 2006. When is quarantine a useful control strategy for emerging infectious diseases? *American Journal of Epidemiology*, 163(5), 479–485. Available online at http://aje.oxfordjournals.org/content/163/5/479.long.

Diallo, B. 2015. *Ebola en Guinee: le Président Condé Utilise l'usage de la « Force » contre les Réticents*. Africaguinee.com, 18 January 2015. Available online at www.africaguinee.com/articles/2015/01/18/ebola-en-guinee-le-president-conde-autorise-l-usage-de-la-force-contre-les.

Diallo, T. and Felix, B. 2014. Mali ends last quarantines, could be Ebola-free next month. *Reuters*, 16 December 2014. Available online at www.reuters.com/article/2014/12/16/us-health-ebola-mali-idUSKBN0JU1NR20141216.

Drazen, J. M., Kanapathipillai, R., Campion, E. W., Rubin, E. J., Hammer, S. M., Morrissey, S. and Baden, L. R. 2014. Ebola and quarantine. *New England Journal of Medicine*, 371(21), 2029–2030. Available online at www.nejm.org/doi/full/10.1056/NEJMe1413139.

Epelboin, A. 2015. *Approche Anthropologique de l' Épidémie de FHV Ebola en Guinée Conakry*. 18 March 2015. Available online at http://memsic.ccsd.cnrs.fr/hal-01090291/document.

Fink, S. 2015. Outbreak. [Documentary]. Frontline. Public Broadcasting Service.

Formenty, P., Libama, F., Epelboin, A., Allarangar, Y., Leroy, E., Moudzeo, H., Tarangonia, P., Molamou, A., Lenzi, M., Ait-Ikhlef, K., Hewlett, B., Roth, C. and Grein, T. 2003. L'épidemie de fièvre hémorragique à virus Ebola en République du Congo, 2003: une nouvelle stratégie? *Médicine Tropale (Mars)*, 63, 291–295.

Garrett, L. 2001. Chapter 2: Landa-landa. In *Betrayal of Trust. The Collapse of Global Public Health*. New York: Hyperion.

Garrett, L. 2014. Heartless but effective: I have seen "cordon sanitaire" work against Ebola. *The New Republic*, 14 August. Available online at www.newrepublic.com/article/119085/ebola-cordon-sanitaire-when-it-worked-congo-1995.

Grigg, C., Waziri, N. E., Olayinka, A. T. and Vertefeuille, J. F. 2015. Use of group quarantine in Ebola control – Nigeria, 2014. *Morbidity and Mortality Weekly Report*, 64(5), 124. Available online at www.cdc.gov/mmwr/preview/mmwrhtml/mm6405a3.htm.

Hewlett, B. S. and Hewlett, B. L. 2008. *Ebola, Culture and Politics: The Anthropology of an Emerging Disease*. Belmont, CA: Thomson Wadsworth.

Hewlett B. L. and Hewlett, B. S. 2005. Providing care and facing death: nursing during Ebola outbreaks in central Africa. *Journal of Transcultural Nursing*, 16(4), 289–297.

Hewlett, B. S., Epelboin, A., Hewlett, B. L. and Formenty, P. 2005. Medical anthropology and Ebola in Congo: cultural models and humanistic care. *Bulletin de la Societe de Pathologie Exotique*, 98(3), 230–236.

Hewlett, B. S. and Amola, R. P. 2003. Cultural contexts of Ebola in Northern Uganda. *Emerging Infectious Diseases*, 9(10), 1242–1248. Available online at wwwnc.cdc.gov/eid/article/9/10/02-0493_article.

Heymann, D. L. 2014. Ebola: learn from the past. *Nature*, 514(7522), 299–300.

Hodge, J. G. Jr, Barraza, L., Measer, G. and Agrawal, A. 2014. Global emergency legal responses to the 2014 Ebola outbreak: public health and the law. *Journal of Law, Medicine and Ethics*, 42(4), 595–601.

Karimova, T. 2015. *Derogation from Human Rights Treaties in Situations of Emergencies*. RULAC project. Geneva: Geneva Academy of International and Humanitarian Law. Available online at http://atlalix.com/project-rulac/issues/derogation-from-human-rights-treaties-in-situations-of-emergency.

Kerstiëns, B. and Matthys, F. 1999. Interventions to control virus transmission during an outbreak of Ebola hemorrhagic fever: experience from Kikwit, Democratic Republic of the Congo, 1995. *Journal of Infectious Diseases*, 179(suppl 1), S263–S267. Available online at http://jid.oxfordjournals.org/content/179/Supplement_1/S263.abstract?sid=2d2d0bd8-3faf-4264-bf50-9e549124d08c.

Koenig, K. L. 2015. Health care worker quarantine for Ebola: to eradicate the virus or alleviate fear? *Annals of Emergency Medicine*, 65(3), 330–331. Available online at www.annemergmed.com/article/S0196-0644%2814%2901571-6/pdf.

Kucharski, A. J., Camacho, A., Flasche, S., Glover, R. E., Edmunds, J. and Funk, S. 2015a. Measuring the impact of Ebola control measures in Sierra Leone. *Proceedings of the National Academy of Sciences of the United States of America*, published ahead of print. Available from: www.pnas.org/content/early/2015/10/07/1508814112.full.pdf?sid=1c78de2e-28e4-497d-9984-223608277f11.

Kucharski, A. J., Camacho, A., Checchi, F., Waldman, R., Grais, R. F., Cabrol, J. C., Briand, S., Baguelin, M., Flasche, S., Funk, S. and Edmunds, W. J. 2015b. Evaluation of the benefits and risks of introducing Ebola community care centers, Sierra Leone. *Emerging Infectious Diseases*, 21(3), 393–399.

Kutalek, R., Wang, S., Fallah, M., Wesseh, C. S. and Gilbert, J. 2015. Ebola interventions: listen to communities. *Lancet*, 3, e131. Available online at www.thelancet.com/pdfs/journals/langlo/PIIS2214-109X%2815%2970010-0.pdf.

Leach, M. and Hewlett B. S. 2010. Haemorrhagic fevers: narratives, politics and pathways. In S. Dry and M. Leach (eds) *Epidemics: Science, Governance and Social Justice* (pp. 43–69). London: Earthscan.

Lyon, G. M., Mehta, A. K., Varkey, J. B., Brantly, K., Plyler, L., McElroy, A. K., Kraft, C. S., Towner, J. S., Spiropoulou, C., Ströher, U., Uyeki, T. M. and Ribner, B. S. 2014. Clinical care of two patients with Ebola virus disease in the United States. *New England Journal of Medicine*, 371(25), 2402–2409. Available online at www.nejm.org/doi/full/10.1056/NEJMoa1409838.

Mac Johnson, R. and Larson, N. 2015. Sierra Leone berates Ebola quarantine escapees as cases surge. *Agence France Presse*, 20 May. Available online at http://reliefweb.int/report/sierra-leone/sierra-leone-berates-ebola-quarantine-escapees-cases-surge.

MacPhail, T. 2014. *The Viral Network. A Pathography of the H1N1 Influenza Pandemic. Chapter 3: Quarantine, Epidemiological Knowledge, and Infectious Disease Research in Hong Kong.* Ithaca, NY, and London: Cornell University Press.

Marais, F., Minkler, M., Gibson, N., Mwau, B., Mehtar, S., Ogunsola, F., Banya, S. S. and Corburn, J. 2015. A community-engaged infection prevention and control approach to Ebola. *Health Promotion International*, 31(2), 440–449. Available online at http:// heapro.oxfordjournals.org/content/early/2015/02/12/heapro.dav003.full.pdf+html.

Maron, D. F. 2015. The most memorable moments of the Ebola response. *Scientific American*, 24 March. Available online at www.youtube.com/watch?feature=player_ embedded&v=vLJPJYy1oN4.

Meltzer, M. I., Atkins, C. Y., Santibanez, S. Knust, B., Petersen, B. W., Ervin, E. D., Nichol, S. T., Damon, I. K. and Washington, M. L. 2014. Estimating the future number of cases in the Ebola epidemic—Liberia and Sierra Leone, 2014–2015. *Morbidity and Mortality Weekly Report*, suppl. 63(3), 1–14. Available online at www.cdc.gov/mmwr/ pdf/other/su6303.pdf.

Merler, S., Ajelli, M., Fumanelli, L., Gomes, M. F. C., Piontti, A. P., Rossi, L., Chao, D. L., Longini, I. M. Jr., Halloran, M. E. and Vespignani, A. 2015. Spatiotemporal spread of the 2014 outbreak of Ebola virus disease in Liberia and the effectiveness of non-pharmaceutical interventions: a computational modelling analysis. *Lancet Infectious Diseases*, 15(2), 204–211. Available online at www.thelancet.com/pdfs/journals/ laninf/PIIS1473-3099%2814%2971074-6.pdf.

Miles, S. U. 2015. Kaci Hickox: public health and the politics of fear. *American Journal of Bioethics*, 15(4), 17–19.

MSF. 2014. *Ebola: Quarantine Can Undermine Efforts to Curb Epidemic.* Press release, 27 October. Available online at www.msf.org/article/ebola-quarantine-can-undermine-efforts-curb-epidemic.

Pandey, A., Atkins, K., Medlock, J., Wenzel, N., Townsend, J. P., Childs, J. E., Nyenswah, T. G., Ndeffo-Mbah, M. L. and Galvani, A. P. 2014. Strategies for containing Ebola in West Africa. *Science*, 346(6212), 991–995. Available online at www.science-mag.org/content/346/6212/991.full.

Presidential Commission for the Study of Bioethical Issues. 2015. *Ethics and Ebola. Public Health Planning and Response. February 2015.* Available online at http:// bioethics.gov/node/4637.

Racaniello, V. 2014. Nobel laureates and Ebola virus quarantine. *Virology Blog*, 4 November 2014. Available online at www.virology.ws/2014/11/04/nobel-laureates-and-ebola-virus-quarantine.

Reliefweb. 2015. *République de Guinée et Organisation Mondiale de la Santé. Rapport de la Situation Epidémiologique Maladie a Virus Ebola en Guinée.* Available online at http://reliefweb.int/updates?search=Rapport%20de%20la%20Situation%20 Epid%C3%A9miologique%20Maladie%20a%20Virus%20Ebola%20en%20 Guin%C3%A9e&page=1#content.

Richards, P., Amara, J., Ferme, M. C., Kamara, P., Mokuwa, E., Sheriff, A. I., Suluku, R. and Voors, M. 2015. Social pathways for Ebola virus disease in rural Sierra Leone, and some implications for containment. *PLoS Neglected Tropical Diseases*, 17, 9(4), e0003567. Available online at http://journals.plos.org/plosntds/article?id=10.1371/ journal.pntd.0003567.

Roddy, P., Weatherill, D., Jeffs, B., Abaakouk, Z., Dorion, C., Rodriguez-Martinez, J., Palma, P. P. de la Rosa, O., Villa, L., Grovas, I. and Borchert, M. 2007. The Médecins Sans Frontières intervention in the Marburg hemorrhagic fever epidemic, Uige, Angola,

2005. II. Lessons learned in the community. *Journal of Infectious Diseases*, 196(suppl. 2), S162–S167. Available online at http://jid.oxfordjournals.org/content/196/Supplement_2/S162.long.

Rothstein, M. A. 2015a. Ebola, quarantine, and the law. *Hastings Center Report*, 45(1), 5–6. Available online at http://onlinelibrary.wiley.com/doi/10.1002/hast.411/pdf.

Rothstein, M. A. 2015b. From SARS to Ebola: legal and ethical considerations for modern quarantine. *Indiana Health Law Review*, 12(1), 227–280.

Rothstein M. A., Alcalde, G. M., Elster, N. R., Majumder, M. A., Palmer, L. I., Stone, H. T. and Hoffman, R. E. 2003. *Quarantine and Isolation: Lessons Learned from SARS. A Report to the Centers for Disease Control and Prevention*. Louisville: Institute for Bioethics, Health Policy and Law, University of Louisville School of Medicine. November 2003. Available online at http://biotech.law.lsu.edu/blaw/cdc/SARS_REPORT.pdf.

Ruble, K. 2014. Ebola riots in Sierra Leone highlight marginalized youth population. *Vice News*, 23 October. Available online at https://news.vice.com/article/ebola-riots-in-sierra-leone-highlight-marginalized-youth-population.

Sahid, J. S. 2015. Pros and cons of Sierra Leone's Ebola lockdowns. *IRIN*, 9 April. Available online at www.irinnews.org/report/101346/ebola-lockdowns-anything-to-get-to-zero.

Shears, P. and O'Dempsey, T. J. D. 2015. Ebola virus disease in Africa: epidemiology and nosocomial transmission. *Journal of Hospital Infection* 90(1), 1–9. Available online at www.journalofhospitalinfection.com/article/S0195-6701%2815%2900046-8/pdf.

Sprecher, A. G, Caluwaerts, A., Draper, M., Feldmann, H., Frey, C. P., Funk, R. H., Kobinger, G., Le Duc, J. W., Spiropoulou, C. and Williams, W. J. 2015. Personal protective equipment for filovirus epidemics: a call for better evidence. *Journal of Infectious Diseases* 212(suppl. 2), S98–S100. Available online at http://jid.oxfordjournals.org/content/early/2015/03/26/infdis.jiv153.long.

Sterk, E. 2008. *Filovirus Haemorrhagic Fever Guideline*. Médecins Sans Frontières.

United Nations. 1985. Siracusa Principles. Human Rights Library. University of Minnesota. Available online at www1.umn.edu/humanrts/instree/siracusaprinciples.html.

Ulrich, C. 2014. Ebola is causing moral distress among African health care workers. *BMJ*, 349, g6672. Available online at www.bmj.com/content/349/bmj.g6672.

USAID. 2015. *Community Perspectives about Ebola in Bong, Lofa and Montserrado Counties of Liberia: results of a qualitative study*. Final report, January 2015. Available online at http://ebolacommunicationnetwork.org/ebolacomresource/community-perspectives-about-ebola-in-bong-lofa-and-montserrado-counties-of-liberia.

Washington, M. L. and Meltzer, M. L. 2015. Effectiveness of Ebola treatment units and community care centers—Liberia, September 23–October 31, 2014. *Morbidity and Mortality Weekly Report*, 63(3), 67–69. Available online at www.cdc.gov/mmwr/preview/mmwrhtml/mm6403a6.htm.

Wilkinson, A. and Leach, M. 2015. Briefing: Ebola—myths, realities and structural violence. *African Affairs (London)*, 114(454), 136–148. Available online at http://afraf.oxfordjournals.org/content/114/454/136.

Witty, C. J. M., Farrar, J., Ferguson, M., Edmunds, W. J., Piot, P., Leach, M. and Davies, S. C. 2014. Infectious disease: tough choices to reduce Ebola transmission. *Nature*, 515(7526), 192–194. Available online at www.nature.com/polopoly_fs/1.16298!/menu/main/topColumns/topLeftColumn/pdf/515192a.pdf.

World Health Organization. 2003. Outbreak(s) of Ebola haemorrhagic fever, Congo and Gabon, October 2001–July 2002. *Weekly Epidemiological Record*, 26, 217–224. Available online at www.who.int/wer/2003/en/wer7826.pdf.

World Health Organization. 2007. *WHO Guidance on Human Rights and Involuntary Detention for xdr-tb Control*. Available online at www.who.int/tb/features_archive/involuntary_treatment/en.

Wynia, M. K. 2007. Ethics and public health emergencies: restrictions on liberty. *American Journal of Bioethics*, 7(2), 1–5.

Zellmann, H. 2015. Counseling through the fence. *TAG*, 39, 23 (internal journal, MSF Switzerland).

7 A history of quarantine

The continued controversy over its legitimacy

Cécile M. Bensimon and Ana Komparic

Introduction

Quarantine is one of the oldest tools of public health. It has been used for centuries, in various capacities, to prevent transmission and stem the tide of communicable disease outbreaks. During the 2003 SARS outbreak, it was invoked on a scale unprecedented in the history of modern public health. In the aftermath, the use of restrictive measures by public health authorities was back on the agenda of policymakers and health care providers in a way that it had not been since the turn of the twentieth century. Every jurisdiction affected by SARS had reached the same conclusion: the only viable way to control the outbreak would be to rely on the centuries-old control measures used in epidemics before the age of bacteriology—contact tracing and follow-up, travel restrictions, isolation, and, most controversially, quarantine. Quarantine has since proven to remain a valid public health strategy in the twenty-first century, even though restricting the movement of healthy persons in modern society is fraught with legal and ethical dilemmas. That it remains an important and contentious public health strategy was reinforced during the 2014 Ebola outbreak, when quarantine was again used on a large scale despite ongoing controversy or outright opposition (Drazen et al., 2014, Barbisch et al., 2015, Koenig, 2015, Rothstein, 2015).

This chapter will describe the history of quarantine, using SARS as a point of reference. The use of quarantine during SARS was the first time that quarantine was used on a large scale in modern public health, that is, since the advent of bacteriology and in an era where rights dominate the moral and legal landscape. It will also point to other modern instances where quarantine was considered but ultimately deemed irrelevant or unnecessary (i.e., HIV/AIDS). The aim of the chapter is to describe the historical progression of the issues raised by the use of quarantine to contextualize the persistent and unresolved issues associated with the use of quarantine during the 2014 Ebola outbreak. Viewed through a historical lens, it will become clear that many fundamental issues associated with the use of quarantine that arose in the past remain relevant today—e.g., multiple interpretations of quarantine, inconsistent applications of quarantine laws across jurisdictional boundaries, claims of ineffectiveness (Barbisch et al., 2015), and the role of the military in enforcing quarantine orders. What is substantively different today is the imperative to respect individual rights and consider the effects of quarantine, an inherently coercive measure, on these rights, thus the raising of the bar to justify limiting rights with "rigorous science" (Koenig, 2015).

Problématique

First introduced as a means to control the infiltration of communicable diseases into local communities, systems of quarantine were originally quasi-institutions commonly erected at seaports that saw thousands of people systematically quarantined at any one time. There was little controversy about its use with respect to the scientific and economic viability of communities. Long before the notion of public health was formulated, both as a discipline and an institution, and even longer before the emphasis on security and protection embodied in the historic conception of the welfare state entered our political consciousness, the use of quarantine was a fundamental pillar of what were essentially public health measures. By all accounts, it was the demands of communicable disease control that drove the development and (re)organization of health systems—so that by the time public health practice came to be known as such, quarantine was already viewed as a necessary and legitimate public health strategy. Quarantine is both one of the oldest tools of—and a precedent to—public health, which was previously viewed as a microcosm of an implicit social contract in which agency was defined in terms of obligations rather than rights.

For nearly half a century, however, when it appeared that communicable diseases were no longer a threat and bacteriology became a respected science, health authorities shifted to surveillance as an alternative to quarantine, fundamentally changing the nature of compulsory public health measures in communicable disease control. Quarantine was no longer the de facto intervention in the control of communicable diseases and was no longer accepted as a valid public health strategy.[1] In effect, it was hardly ever, if at all, considered to be a viable option—much less so when invoked on a large scale such as when SARS emerged globally in February 2003.[2]

The emergence and re-emergence of communicable diseases—such as SARS and Ebola, MDR- and XDR-TB (multi-drug-resistant and extensively drug-resistant tuberculosis), and catastrophic public health emergencies such as the 2004 Asian Tsunami and Hurricane Katrina in 2006—have given rise to a renewed imperative to focus on the fundamental importance of public health policies (see, for example, Coker, 2001; Gostin, 2000; National Advisory Committee of SARS and Public Health, 2003; Markel, 2005; World Health Organization, 2006; SARS Commission and Campbell, 2006; Allan et al., 2007; Bloomberg, 2007; Fidler et al., 2007). These crises highlighted how public health plays an instrumental role in securing the conditions necessary for people to be healthy and in shaping the development and outcomes of communicable disease outbreaks or other emergencies. In particular, the SARS and Ebola outbreaks demonstrated that the exercise of quarantine powers raises fundamental issues about the use of restrictive measures, acting as a "gravitational pull" that engages and connects broader political, governance, legal (Fidler, 2004; Fidler et al., 2007, p. 616), and ethical issues.

The society in which quarantine was invoked during the SARS and Ebola outbreaks is fundamentally different than the world in which it was first conceived and enforced. Historically, quarantine was deemed to be a societal good bearing a moral clout that *obligated* individuals to abide by restrictive measures (Fidler, 1999, pp. 170–179). Today, citizens naturally presuppose that they have the *right* not to adhere to autonomy-limiting measures, even if they comply with them—a view which reflects a deeply entrenched mode of public thinking that can be described in Kymlicka's (2002, p. 7) terms as the development of a "rights consciousness"[3] in which questions of rights are questions of basic morality.

In essence, the exercise of quarantine powers raises deep questions concerning the role and nature of public health in modern society and the challenges it poses to individual rights. Given this, the history of quarantine can best be understood through the lens of the institutionalization of public health, while the challenges raised by its continued use can be appreciated through the lens of the relationship between individual rights and public health, tied as it is to questions of the common good.

The institutionalization of public health: the dominance of disease control

The Institute of Medicine (1988, p. 19) states that "Public health is what we, as a society, do collectively to assure the conditions of people to be healthy."[4] As Gostin (2001, p. 122) suggests, the richness of this definition can be "appreciated by examining its constituent parts." He comments:

> The emphasis on cooperative and mutually shared obligations ("we, as a society") reinforces the collective entities (e.g. governments and communities) take responsibility for healthy populations ... there is a great deal individuals cannot do to secure their health; to overcome whatever these barriers may be, individuals need to organize, work together, and share their resources. Acting alone, people cannot achieve environmental protection, hygiene and sanitation, clean air and surface water, uncontaminated food and drinking water, safe roads and products, and control of communicable disease. Each of these collective goods, and many more, is achievable only by organized and sustained community activities.
>
> (Gostin, 2001, p. 123)

We can appreciate Gostin's observations by understanding these in the historical context of public health's emergence as a response to the problems (relating to food, water, sanitation, and disease) created by communal living in newly urbanized or urbanizing centres. The rise of urban living led to a new (health and social) imperative: that of providing the conditions necessary for the development and sustainability of communities. As towns and cities emerged, the responsibility for providing basic provisions for healthy living could no longer be left to individual or private business interests, and what would essentially become public health measures appeared in the nineteenth century (Encyclopaedia of Bioethics, 2004, p. 2157). These measures were strategically carried out by the state, which began taking responsibility for the prevention of disease through organized and sustained community activities. The recognition that public health required a more comprehensive system for civic sanitation, among other things, generated myriad initiatives that eventually shaped public health organization into a more systematic and integrated discipline, ultimately leading to the institutionalization of modern public health as a vehicle of collective action that both creates and guarantees the conditions necessary to a life in common.

The history of public health is inextricably tied to the history of communicable disease control and, specifically, quarantine as the first method used for the prevention and containment of epidemics. Public health measures to control communicable diseases had been instituted long before—and in fact significantly contributed to—the institutionalization of public health. Since the prevention and treatment of disease was a necessary presupposition to communal living, it is easy to see how that would be the case.

Quarantine

Historically speaking,[5] the concept of quarantine precedes modern notions of public health. Concern over, and the practice of, isolating persons with communicable diseases and corresponding sanitary procedures can be traced back to the Old Testament, where one can find detailed instructions in the Books of Leviticus and Numbers for the treatment of lepers (Rothstein et al., 2003, p. 17). Other early recordings that urged the use of such formalized practices date back to Thucydides (*c*.460–400 BCE), Hippocrates (*c*.460–370 BCE), and Galen of Pergamon (*c*.130–200 CE). Medical historians report that one of the earliest known uses of quarantine to control the movement of travelers from regions of the world where the plague was known to be spreading was enacted in 532 CE by the Byzantine emperor Justinian, who ordered that travelers and sailors be "cleansed" in special facilities before entering the city of Constantinople (Markel, 1997, p. 3; Rothstein et al., 2003, p. 17). Similar practices that were used over succeeding centuries have been documented in seventh-century China and other parts of Asia, as well as in Europe during the Middle Ages.

The concept of quarantine (in Italian *quarantina* and *quaranta giorni*) was first construed in the fourteenth century by Venetian officials, referring to a 40-day period during which ships entering the Port of Venice were required to remain in isolation before any person or merchandise was permitted ashore. In 1374, Venice enacted a 40-day quarantine regulation, and in 1403 it instituted the first formal system of quarantine, imposing the isolation and detention of all ships. This Venetian model held sway and was reproduced around the globe, from the fourteenth through the nineteenth century, as the spread of epidemics intensified owing to the rise of international travel and commerce during and following the Renaissance. As Markel (1997, p. 3) observes,

> from medieval times on, shutting the gates of a city or port to all those suspected of being ill and isolating those sick people discovered to have entered represented the best, and often the only, means available for stemming the tide of an epidemic.

The practice of preventing entry of contagion into a city was known as a cordon sanitaire ("sanitary cordon"), a geographic quarantine formed by a ring of armed soldiers guarding the gates of the city.[6]

During the nineteenth century, contemporaneous health organizations were not yet systematic enough to effectively control the spread of epidemics—which only seemed to be proliferating, spanning from the plague to yellow fever and cholera by the mid-1800s. The devastating impact of these later epidemics galvanized international interest, especially by European nations with commercial or colonial interests, to establish an international board of sanitary or quarantine control, leading, in 1851, to the first of a series of international sanitary conferences that continued for the better part of the twentieth century (Markel, 1997, p. 4).

For decades, however, no meaningful consensus on international control of communicable diseases was reached, in large part, explain Rothstein et al. (2003, p. 18), "because of the political bickering between European powers with competing interests in preserving or enlarging their commerce and trade with the Middle East and Asia." Yet, as bacteriology became more and more accepted, and as major diseases such as typhoid and cholera were attributed to specific germs, delegates began to agree on rudimentary measures for containment and control by the 1890s. As a result, "substantive consensus on international sanitary and quarantine regulations began to emerge" (Stern and Markel, 2004, p. 1476), leading to the signing of the first International Sanitary Convention at the Seventh Sanitary Conference in 1892. Notably, the Eleventh Sanitary Conference led to the establishment of the first permanent international health organization, the International Office of Public Hygiene (IOPH), a precursor to the World Health Organization, which was established as the world's chief public health organization following World War II.

This century-long focus on communicable diseases in international diplomacy and international law ultimately led to the harmonization of national quarantine regulations, as well as the creation of an international communicable disease surveillance system instituting a rather sophisticated international system of quarantine by the end of the nineteenth century.

By then, the maritime definition of quarantine had changed markedly from its medieval origins, no longer being based on the 40-day period of detention. As the international sanitary conferences began to exert greater authority on international communicable disease control, and as bacteriology's tenets began to dominate public health and medicine, the precise definition and length of quarantine began to vary widely, depending on the location and specificity of a particular disease and the understanding of physicians of that era[7] (Cumming, 1921).

This differentiation of quarantine measures engendered a systematic integration of quarantine measures into medical practice, or what Gensini et al. (2004, p. 260) call a "deep medicalization of quarantine" during the late nineteenth century. Supported by a well-developed system of medical inspection and detention, the treatment of those admitted to the isolation hospital at quarantine stations was largely supportive and no longer punitive, as had been the case when quarantine was first instituted. This trend towards a "medicalized" quarantine essentially served to reinforce the notion that it was a valid strategy for communicable disease control.

As Markel (1997) observes, it is tempting to view the history of quarantine as one without controversy from the distance of a century of events. Although it was indeed strengthened and reinforced as a viable practice over time, there was widespread opposition to quarantines throughout the nineteenth century,[8] which crystallized by the beginning of the twentieth century as scientific and technological developments began reshaping the international health landscape. First and foremost, arguments against quarantine focused on its nefarious impact on trade and property interests, leading many observers to argue against the questionable effectiveness of traditional quarantine measures. Hancock (1821, p. 237) captured this line of thinking in 1821, arguing that:

> Without being so secure a defence as is commonly imagined, quarantine establishments have been maintained with multiplied inconveniences and hardships; and that we are more indebted to chance than good management for our preservation; it's high time we should know whether they be essential or not; whether they not be a mere form; and whether it would not be safer to dispense with them entirely, than to rely for security on burthensome regulations defectively administered, which oppress whilst they deceive.

Later advances in technologies of communication and transportation, which led to an exponential growth in international trade, put great pressure on medical authorities to limit quarantine regulations that were thought to burden its flow. In fact, Fidler (1999) notes that efforts undertaken to harmonize quarantine regulations were merely a strategy for reducing the burdens on European trade created by national disease control measures. The view that quarantine posed unnecessary and "vexatious" (Forster 1832, p. 4) obstacles to commerce was further exacerbated by the wide spectrum of beliefs about the etiology of communicable diseases.

Throughout the early history of communicable disease control, quarantines were often devised even by those who did not believe in the existence of germs; they used quarantine not as a means of biological containment but as a broad and perverse means of isolating undesirable social groups (historically, the

poor, the disenfranchised, and immigrants). Markel (1997, p. 4) skilfully illustrates, through his exploration of the social, cultural, medical, and political
issues surrounding the quarantine of East European Jewish immigrants during
the typhus and cholera epidemics of New York City in 1892, that "one of the
strongest leitmotifs in the history of epidemics and quarantines in the US is the
use of quarantine as a medical rationale to isolate and stigmatize social groups
reviled for other reasons."

Even though New York's National Quarantine Act of 1893 recognized and
warned against the conflation of communicable disease control and social
scapegoating by stating that "policies of isolation and quarantine to protect the
public health should be a function separate from that of the control or restriction of immigration" (Markel, 1997, p. 190), many reproached that quarantine
measures arbitrarily targeted undesirable persons and thus interfered arbitrarily
with civic liberties. Such opposition from those who believed that quarantines
were used by the state for purposes other than disease control remained widespread, giving rise to the view that disease control had to be "tailored narrowly
to public health needs so as not to interfere arbitrarily with individual freedom"
(Fidler, 1999, p. 170).

It was in this context that formal claims against public health measures on the
grounds of (some notions of) individual liberty began appearing in the courts,
planting the seeds of future constitutional challenges. Initially, however, arguments against quarantine focused on trade and property interests rather than on
any serious concern for the rights of individuals.[9] In the context of communicable disease control, there was both a limited definition of—and limited concern
for—rights because individuals did not possess "a set of well-defined rights that
could be weighed against conflicting social needs"[10] (Merritt, 1986a, p. 4). Thus,
the courts' invariable response was to "strongly endorse the power of the state
and local governments to adopt stringent measures controlling disease" (Merritt,
1986a, p. 3). This was consistent with the prevailing view that systems of quarantine were a microcosm of the then-prevalent social contract, according to
which individuals' rights were subordinate to "the higher rights of the community" (Fox, 1986, p. 13), and that public health was "the highest law of the
land" (Merritt, 1986a, p. 13). The protection of public health, and with it the
implicit obligation to comply with control measures, thus continued to take precedence over rights—even in the United States of America, whose constitution
provided strong protections for individual liberties and civil and political rights.

The oft-cited case of *Jacobson v. Massachusetts*, decided in 1905 by the US
Supreme Court, set an important precedent in recognizing that public health
supersedes individual rights—in fact, it laid the foundation for public health
law in the US—when Jacobson challenged the constitutionality of Massachusetts's immunization law and refused to be vaccinated against smallpox. It was
the first time that the US Supreme Court considered an individual's claim that
a compulsory public health measure violated his "inherent right" to liberty,
marking the beginning of a transition towards the recognition of rights in
public health. Yet, while the US Supreme Court agreed to consider Jacobson's

constitutional arguments against compulsory public health measures, it effectively rejected each argument, ruling that the

> liberty secured by the Constitution of the United States to every person within its jurisdiction does not import an absolute right in each person to be, at all times and in all circumstances, wholly freed from restraint. There are manifold restraints to which every person is necessarily subject for the common good.
>
> (*Jacobson v. Massachusetts*, 1905)

The Supreme Court affirmed the right of states to enforce public health measures as a legitimate use of public health's police powers, clearly reinforcing that the protection of public health outweighed individual rights.

Thus, in the early history of public health, state involvement was viewed as leading to positive consequences—in effect drawing on the strength of the justificatory power of public health's utilitarian pursuit. Public health was a means to redress the fundamental problems caused by the devastating health effects of communal living and the natural tendency of private interests to fail to extend services to all segments of society (such as the poor). It was generally accepted that public health endeavours increased general welfare, granting it a privileged authority. Individuals had obligations, not rights, especially when it came to communicable disease control (Fidler, 1999, pp. 170–179). Even where formal claims of individual rights were made against public health measures, public health predominantly trumped individual rights (Fidler, 1999). But the notion that individual liberty invariably yields to public health would change radically.

The institutionalization of human rights: disease control and human rights

The rise of rights

As scientific and technological developments began reshaping the international health landscape at the turn of the twentieth century, the view that individuals had obligations and not rights in public health changed. With the rise of bacteriology, quarantine was becoming less acceptable as a public health strategy; so was the broader role of public health, which was increasingly viewed as paternalistic and intrusive. At least in the United States, this sentiment became manifest in the courts, which showed a greater willingness to challenge and invalidate public health measures, a trend that intensified by 1940 with the replacement of a *negative* view of individual rights with a *positive* one (Merritt, 1986a).

By applying this new definition of rights, the courts recognized that individuals retained a set of fundamental rights that could, in some circumstances, legitimately override public health interests if a health risk was deemed insufficient to outweigh the burden on individual rights (Merritt, 1986a, p. 8). This repositioning represented a radical departure from the view that even constitutionally guaranteed rights must invariably yield to the demands of communicable disease control. More importantly, it paved the way for a paradigm shift in public health discourse and practice that recognized that individuals have rights in the context of public health, particularly in the context of communicable disease control.

What crystallized this shift, however, was what we can aptly call the human rights revolution. The disclosure and eventual reporting of the atrocities that took place in Nazi concentration camps galvanized a humanitarian movement that sought to create conditions that would prevent such atrocities in the future. It is reasonable to speak of a "revolution" in thinking about the impact that this movement had, as it ultimately led to the institutionalization of human rights norms in international law. While there is a long history behind human rights thinking, the human rights revolution effectively constitutionalized the Kantian idea that all people *necessarily* possess equal and absolute rights that are inherent to them *simply because they are human.*

The institutionalization of human rights has had profound implications for society: The view that individual rights have independent, positive weights, and weights of different value, *fundamentally* transformed the notion and status of rights in modern society, and in so doing it redefined the social contract between the state and the individual by reversing the public health tradition that emphasized individual duties and obligations rather than rights and freedoms. In turn, the explicit emphasis on human rights saw the entrenchment of two notions that had faint precursors in American jurisprudence and early British and Canadian sanitary reforms. First, it engendered greater scrutiny of public health measures that interfered with individual rights, such as the use of quarantine, and, second, government responsibility for providing conditions conducive to public health was positively established (Fidler, 1999, pp. 170–179, Merritt, 1986b). These developments made explicit the intersection of human rights and disease control, thereby weaving a new social fabric that explicitly recognized that "[v]irtually every measure of disease control has human rights implications" (Tomasevski et al., 1992, p. 539).

At first, the linkage between public health and human rights, which aimed to balance the exigencies of the protection of public health against the protection of individual rights, formally sanctioned the use of restrictive measures under conditions of threat to the public health and recognized public health as a legitimate pursuit even in the context of the institutionalization of rights (Siracusa Principles, 1984). But this would all change during the HIV/AIDS debate.

The HIV/AIDS debate: bringing human rights to bear on public health

If we go back to the last major debate on communicable disease control before SARS emerged, the prospect of quarantine quickly became an explosive issue when it was resurrected from the annals of public health in the early 1980s during the HIV/AIDS crisis. When public attention and health officials turned to quarantine at the dawn of the crisis, some going as far as drafting regulations to respond to what was taken to be a matter of serious public concern, the renewed interest in quarantine spurred an intense and often passionate debate on the impact of the use of restrictive measures on the rights of victims or carriers of HIV/AIDS (see for example, Novick, 1985; Parmet, 1985–1986; Gostin and Curran, 1986; Macklin, 1986; Fox, 1986; Merritt, 1986a, 1986b; Ford and Quam, 1987; Bayer and Fairchild-Carrino, 1993; Mann et al., 1994). Growing concerns over the return, or even just the prospect of a return, to traditional restrictive public health measures pioneered a human rights approach to public health that many say was "one of the most important and unanticipated outcomes of the first decade of the AIDS pandemic" (Mann, 1992, p. 537). Foremost, it was a catalyst for beginning to define some of the structural connections between health and human rights, with a view to protecting what was thought to be most at stake in communicable disease control: the paramount value of human well-being and dignity.

In practical terms, the HIV/AIDS debate sharpened the focus of the public health/human rights discourse by raising two interrelated issues: the lack of regard for modern notions of due process procedures in public health law, and the need to modernize the provisions of the International Health Regulations that guided public health measures, which had not been updated to incorporate human rights norms. Thus it was that the HIV/AIDS debate "brought the human rights revolution to bear on public health" (Fidler, 1999, p. 198), for, as Tomasevski et al. (1992, p. 538) noted, it was "the first worldwide epidemic to occur in the modern era of human rights."

In a review of public health statutes in American states, Gostin and Lazzarini (1997, p. 20) noted that most American legal and public health scholars found that "most state communicable disease statutes fail to ensure [modern notions of] due process procedures for exercising public health powers." They concluded that even countries that respected civil and political rights had yet to reform public health laws to bring them into conformity with human rights norms. Moreover, the International Health Regulations (IHRs) on communicable disease control were limited to provisions for yellow fever, cholera, and plague (Siracusa Principles, 1984). While some argued that the relevance to other communicable diseases could be found in the regulations' assertion that the use of restrictive measures ought to be applied when it is "epidemiologically necessary," just what that actually meant was unclear even in the context of yellow fever, cholera, and plague.

It was further concluded that the use of other restrictive measures against carriers or victims of HIV/AIDS would have the perverse effect of discouraging people from seeking treatment and counselling. The National Academy of Sciences (1986, p. 126) captured this line of thinking, stating that "coercive programs may not only be ineffectual, they may actually undermine individuals' sense of responsibility for the community [and] would be ineffective, if not counterproductive in altering the course of the epidemic." For this reason, it was believed that a voluntaristic approach that respected the rights of individuals with HIV/AIDS would be more effective than traditional, compulsory infection control strategies (Gostin and Curran, 1986, p. 24; Bayer, 1991). "Respecting human rights," stated Gostin and Lazzarini (1997, p. 538), "was the surest way to encourage people to participate in public health programs that offer testing, counselling, education, partner notification, and treatment." As such, public health and human rights were conceived as a continuum wherein the protection and promotion of rights was critical to the protection and promotion of public health.

Bayer and Fairchild (2004, p. 478) aptly summarize the conclusions of the HIV/AIDS debate: "A simple dictum emerged: No public health policy that violated the rights of individuals could be effective in controlling the spread of HIV." In turn, Gruskin and Tarantola (2002) emphasized the importance of the dialogue between public health and human rights pioneered through the debate on HIV/AIDS, stating that the

> groundbreaking contribution of this era lies in the recognition of the applicability of international law to HIV/AIDS issues and in the attention this approach then generated to the linkages between other health issues and human rights – and therefore the ultimate responsibility and accountability of the state under international law for issues relating to health and well-being.
>
> (Gruskin and Tarantola, 2002, p. 1)

The HIV/AIDS debate fundamentally questioned the purpose and boundaries of public health. The rights discourse moved away from the question of weighing rights against public health and instead sought to align human rights principles with public health measures. Thereupon, the linkage was more substantive: human rights activists and scholars alike challenged the prevailing view that human rights and public health are fundamentally in conflict and argued that they are complementary approaches to the common objective of addressing and advancing human well-being. Based on this logic, the protection of rights was seen as an effective public health strategy and, for this reason, it was thought that "public health endeavours should begin and end with a respect for human rights" (de Gordon, Centers and Diovaldes, 1993, p. 1426).

The HIV/AIDS debate over health and human rights essentially reversed the linkage between rights and public health established in early human rights jurisprudence by shifting the focus from the imperative of weighing rights *against public health considerations* to weighing public health *against rights protections* (see, for example, Gostin, 2000; Harris and Martin, 2004; Coker, 2001, 2006). Human rights activists and scholars vehemently opposed the use of quarantine, an "archaic doctrine" (Parmet 1985–1986), and argued that it was unjustified on scientific, legal, or ethical grounds. Over time, most people accepted the new prevailing view that education was the best, and perhaps only, acceptable response (see, for example, Bayer and Dupuis, 1995; Asch et al., 1998).

The legacy of the HIV/AIDS debate was deeply significant. It pioneered a human rights approach to public health that championed human rights as the bedrock of legitimacy for public health practice. Most people believed that the union of human rights and public health would have broader policy implications, and that future public health practice—especially in the context of communicable disease control—would embrace a human rights agenda and "would face human rights scrutiny" (Fidler, 2000, p. 198), especially in the United States, where rights discourse had gained a stronghold in public health practice (see, for example, New York City Tuberculosis Working Group, 1992).

The 2014 Ebola outbreak: revisiting quarantine in the human rights era

The continued controversy

The legacy of the human rights approach to public health has proven to be less straightforward. Arguments against the use of restrictive measures for victims or carriers of HIV/AIDS drew much of their strength from the fact that HIV/AIDS is not analogous to diseases for which quarantine had traditionally been used, such as plague, typhoid, cholera, or even tuberculosis (see for example Bayer, 1991). Similarly, the dynamic nature of today's emerging and re-emerging communicable diseases—such as Ebola, SARS, and XDR-TB—is not analogous to HIV/AIDS, challenging the primacy of rights protections in public health for diseases with different and more pervasive means of transmission than HIV/AIDS.

Yet the question of how to control communicable disease outbreaks in modern society was essentially taken out of the HIV/AIDS debate. Thus, in practical terms, public health had no modern precedent on which to base decisions for the use of quarantine until SARS (as discussed in the problématique) and, most recently, Ebola. It is in the shadow of the urgent dilemmas that confronted public health authorities during the SARS and Ebola outbreaks that the exigencies of disease control and the human rights impact of restrictive public health policy instruments, such as quarantine, revived the conflict between individual rights and public health protections and reignited the debate about the use of quarantine.

Quarantine in the 2014 Ebola outbreak

Debate about the legitimacy of quarantine as a public health measure came to a head during the 2014 West African Ebola outbreak, which saw the first use of mass quarantine and cordons sanitaires in the human rights era.[11] Identified in rural Guinea in March 2014, the Ebola outbreak spread rapidly to urban centres and neighbouring Liberia and Sierra Leone. Peaking in late 2014, but persisting until 2016, the outbreak resulted in over 28,000 infections and more than 11,000 deaths (Emrick et al., 2016). Transmission accelerated rapidly in mid-2014 as traditional public health measures such as contact tracing and surveillance failed. Early efforts to isolate symptomatic individuals and quarantine exposed individuals were unsuccessful owing to weak health systems, scarce health care resources and facilities, and insufficient support and incentives for individuals to adhere to quarantine orders (e.g., failure to provide basic necessities such as food, water, and health care)[12] (Koch, 2015; Thompson, 2016).

On August 1, 2016, as fear intensified amid increasing transmission, failing health systems, and a tepid international response, Guinea, Liberia, and Sierra Leone announced mass quarantines in the tri-border area at the centre of the epidemic, with military personnel closing internal roads and borders in an attempt to contain the outbreak (McNeill, 2014). Shortly after, the Liberian president instituted a cordon sanitaire, enforced by armed soldiers in riot gear, around Monrovia's West Point neighborhood, effectively trapping its 75,000 residents without warning (Greene, 2015). This quarantine, which would become the most publicized instance of military enforcement in the outbreak, was lifted after 10 days as opposition by residents and violent clashes with the military left one civilian dead and several seriously injured. Mass quarantines were instituted on other occasions in Guinea, Liberia, and Sierra Leone, while cordons sanitaires were used in Liberia and Guinea (Hodge et al., 2014).

The use of quarantine received much attention, but, unlike with HIV/AIDS, there was broad acknowledgment that the use of liberty-restricting measures may be permissible to limit Ebola transmission if scientifically warranted and respectful of human rights (Eba, 2014; Hodge et al., 2014; Barbisch et al., 2015; Silva and Smith, 2015; Thompson, 2016). Criticism stemmed from the fact that at least some of the quarantines and cordons sanitaires implemented during the Ebola outbreak failed to meet these conditions. Writing about the widespread use of coercive liberty-restricting measures during the 2014 Ebola outbreak, Eba (2014, p. 2092) asserted that

> such measures violate the rights to liberty and security. In some countries, restrictions to freedom of movement are leading to further human rights violations and humanitarian crises, since people in quarantined zones cannot always access food, health care, or other services.

Moreover, the quarantines, including the West Point cordon sanitaire, were denounced as "unscientific" and not epidemiologically warranted (Thompson, 2016, p. 9) as they restricted asymptomatic individuals, including those who had not been in contact with infected individuals, and even risked exacerbating transmission (Towers et al., 2014). Governments were criticized for failing to provide those under quarantine with necessary supportive measures and for the lack of transparency around decision-making, which bred mistrust in government officials as well as public health authorities and medical providers (Eba, 2014; Thompson, 2016).

Looking forward: the place of quarantine and the role of the military

The 2003 SARS and 2014 Ebola outbreaks suggest that quarantine will likely be invoked in the future to stem the transmission of highly contagious or virulent communicable diseases. While the debate over the legitimacy of quarantine is far from settled, some consensus has emerged from the 2014 Ebola epidemic concerning the use of quarantine and military enforcement. Although the examples of SARS and Ebola suggest that human rights and individual liberties are not trumps over public health, the rise of human rights has shaped the conditions under which quarantine may be considered a legitimate public health practice.

The Ebola outbreak is instructive for future epidemics that may warrant quarantine, including in humanitarian interventions. First and foremost, there is broad agreement that quarantine should only be used when it is the least restrictive possible measure and is proportionate to the risk being mitigated (Silva and Smith, 2015; Thompson, 2016). An additional condition, which was elaborated following SARS but became even more significant in the Ebola response, is reciprocity. That is, when people have their liberties curtailed to protect public health, the public—usually through governments—has reciprocal obligations to those who are quarantined (e.g., to ensure access to basic necessities such as food, water, and health care, as well as compensation for lost income), rather than allowing a disease to run its course in quarantined areas, as is often the case in a cordon sanitaire (Silva and Smith, 2015; Thompson, 2016). Beyond protecting human rights, supportive measures are required to ensure the viability of quarantines by enabling individuals to respect quarantine orders. It has even been suggested that reciprocity should extend beyond an outbreak to include obligations with respect to the side effects of liberty-restricting measures incurred by individuals and communities (Silva and Smith, 2015).[13] Furthermore, transparent communication about the purpose and nature of quarantine measures is crucial to engendering trust and minimizing conflict between civilians and those enforcing the quarantine (Eba, 2014; Greene, 2015; Thompson, 2016).

Military enforcement of quarantines during the Ebola outbreak also received a great deal of critical attention.[14] On the one hand, national militaries and police forces were called upon to enforce quarantines in the affected areas. Referencing the West Point cordon sanitaire, Greene (2015, p. 68) describes the conditions under which mass quarantines may be invoked even in the face of scientific opposition:

> Some events, particularly those that generate the kind of fear associated with the threat of war and pandemic disease, carry an irresistible momentum with them—a momentum that propels people to take action, often with a desperation that will not allow for cool reflection or regard for historical precedent. When a nation feels that kind of profound fear, it often calls upon its military.

Yet, Eba (2014, p. 2092) captures a common concern about the erosion of public trust following the widespread use of military-enforced quarantines, warning that "[t]he deployment of military troops to enforce mass quarantine in such an environment of mistrust might reinforce defiance and further alienate people who must be engaged in the response to Ebola."

On the other hand, foreign military personnel were deployed to support humanitarian and medical missions in response to the Ebola outbreak after a lagging international response prompted Médecins Sans Frontières (MSF) to appeal for foreign military intervention on the grounds that militaries were able to mobilize quickly and extensively (Kamradt-Scott et al., 2015). However, MSF and others stressed that foreign military involvement should be limited to supportive capacities and not the enforcement of quarantines (Eba, 2014; Thompson, 2016). There are also indications that foreign military presence was key to convincing NGOs to remain or establish operations in West Africa during the outbreak (Kamradt-Scott et al., 2015), which raises questions about the legitimacy of foreign militaries acting as security forces in humanitarian interventions. Whether or not humanitarian organizations, and even foreign militaries, can legitimately implement and enforce coercive liberty-restricting measures in the absence of functioning health systems and governments during a public health emergency remains unclear (Thompson, 2016).

Foreign military involvement in the Ebola outbreak also raised questions about the quarantine of military personnel. For example, the US instituted policies to quarantine returning humanitarian and military personnel for 21 days despite criticism that quarantining asymptomatic individuals was not a scientifically warranted restriction of civil liberties (Drazen et al., 2014; Lane and McNair, 2015; Koenig, 2015; Thompson, 2016). Moreover, Lane and McNair (2015) note that, while humanitarian volunteers were vocal about their rights infringements, military personnel do not have the liberty to choose or question deployment, raising questions about whether the duty to serve persists in epidemics. Some countries, like the US, instituted quarantine measures for asymptomatic individuals from affected areas, including for aid and medical workers and military personnel deployed to West Africa (Emrick et al., 2016), while others, including Canada and Australia, instituted "defensive" quarantines by restricting entry and immigration from affected countries (Koch, 2015; Emrick et al., 2016). Moreover, defensive quarantine measures were sometimes justified using a military rationale (Koch, 2015)—where liberties can be curtailed in times of war—challenging a human rights approach to communicable disease control.

The use of mass quarantine in the 2014 Ebola epidemic reinforced the view that public health responses to communicable disease outbreaks must take account of individual rights and prevent human rights abuses. Additionally, the military's role in enforcing liberty-restricting measures was questioned, especially insofar as it damaged public trust, which is essential to effective public health responses. Nonetheless, quarantine was recognized as a possible tool for communicable disease control. This raises further difficult questions about what constitutes a legitimate use of restrictive measures and what ought to be the scope of the military or humanitarian response to communicable disease outbreaks—e.g., which rights take precedence on an international level? Who has the legitimacy to enforce restrictive measures? What types of restrictive measures can be imposed on humanitarian and military personnel? Such questions merit future exploration, for, as history suggests, it is only a matter of time before the prospect of quarantine resurfaces in the context of another epidemic.

Notes

1 We recognize that public health includes environmental health, whereby animals and plants are regularly quarantined as a means to avoid introducing or spreading disease. For the purpose of this inquiry, however, we are limiting the scope of quarantine to human persons.
2 For a detailed description, see Rothstein et al. (2003).
3 Briefly, rights consciousness developed from the liberal assumption that rights are prior to the (common) good and, from this, it follows that rights constitute the basis for determining the justifiability of public health interventions.
4 This definition is the most-cited contemporary definition of public health.
5 We owe much of the following overview to Howard Markel, who gives a rich account of the history of quarantine, which is based largely on his original research in Markel (1997).
6 The use of checkpoints for examining and disinfecting vehicles and persons crossing jurisdictions during SARS was referred by some as cordons sanitaires (Rothstein et al., 2003, p. 129).
7 In reality, as Markel (1997, p. 7) notes, the health officer could legally set the detention for any period of isolation he decreed, regardless of the opinions or theories of others.
8 Opposition could even turn violent, as was the case with civilian opposition to a military-enforced mass quarantine instituted in Munchie, Indiana, in 1893 in response to a smallpox outbreak (Greene, 2015).
9 Merritt (1986a, p. 5) notes that at the time "judges were particularly inclined to invalidate public health measures when they happened to interfere with business operations."
10 Conceptions of rights were limited to the notion of negative rights, according to which persons have the right to pursue their own ends insofar as they do not harm others. Berlin (1969, p. 153) ably summarizes this conception of negative liberty:

> Most modern liberals, at their most consistent, want a situation in which as many individuals as possible can realize as many of their ends as possible, without assessment of the value of these ends as such, save insofar as they may frustrate the purposes of others.

11 Quarantines were used in several communicable disease outbreaks in the latter half of the twentieth century (e.g., the 1972 smallpox outbreak in Yugoslavia (Bhatnagar et al., 2006) and the 1995 Ebola outbreak in Zaire (Heymann, 2014), neither of which was a democracy at the time), but the outbreaks were contained and the quarantines received limited publicity internationally.
12 Conversely, other countries where Ebola spread, including Nigeria, Mali, and Senegal, managed to swiftly contain Ebola, at least in part owing to superior health and laboratory facilities, rigorous contact tracing paired with monitoring and isolation, and effective public education and community engagement (World Health Organization, 2015).
13 For example, Silva and Smith (2015) suggest that compensation may be necessary to remedy long-term disadvantage, such as to farms and businesses that were destroyed as a result of mass quarantines in the tri-border area during the 2014 Ebola outbreak.
14 This chapter limits the discussion of the military in relation to quarantine, but the broader role of the military and civil–military relations during the 2014 Ebola outbreak has been examined elsewhere (see for example Khoshdel, 2014; Greene, 2015; Kamradt-Scott et al., 2015; Lane and McNair, 2015).

References

Allan, S. M., Meier, B. M., Miles, J., Underheim, G. and Haddix, A. C. 2007. Why and how states are updating their public health laws. *The Journal of Law, Medicine & Ethics*, 35(4), 39–42.

Asch, S., Leake, B., Anderson, R. and Gelberg, L. 1998. Why do symptomatic patients delay obtaining care for tuberculosis? *American Journal of Respiratory and Critical Care Medicine*, 157, 1244–1248.

Barbisch, D., Koeniga, K. L. and Shiha, F.-Y. 2015. Is there a case for quarantine? Perspectives from SARS to Ebola. *Disaster Medicine and Public Health Preparedness*, 9(5), 547–553.

Bayer, R. 1991. Public health policy and the AIDS epidemic: an end to HIV exceptionalism? *New England Journal of Medicine*, 324, 1500–1504.

Bayer, R. and Dupuis, L. 1995. Tuberculosis, public health, and civil liberties. *Annual Review of Public Health*, 16, 307–326.

Bayer, R. and Fairchild-Carrino, A. 1993. AIDS and the limits of control: public health orders, quarantine, and recalcitrant behavior. *American Journal of Public Health*, 83(10), 1471–1476.

Bayer, R, and Fairchild, A. L. 2004. The genesis of public health ethics. *Bioethics*, 18(6), 473–492.

Berlin, Isaiah (1969) Two concepts of liberty. In I. Berlin, *Four Essays on Liberty*. Oxford: Oxford University Press.

Bhatnagar, V. Stoto, M. A., Morton, S. C., Boer, R. and Bozzette, S. A. 2006. Transmission patterns of smallpox: systematic review of natural outbreaks in Europe and North America since World War II. *BMC Public Health*, 6, 126.

Bloomberg, M. R. 2007. New public health strategies for a new era. *The Journal of Law, Medicine & Ethics*, 35(4), 28–32.

Coker, R. 2001. Civil liberties and public good: detention of tuberculosis patients and the Public Health Act 1984. *Medical History*, 45(3), 341–358.

Coker, R. and Martin, R. 2006. Introduction: the importance of law for public health policy and practice. *Public Health*, 120(S1), 2–7.

Cumming, H. S. 1921. *The United States Quarantine System during the Past Fifty Years: A Half Century of Public Health*. New York: American Public Health Association.

de Gordon, A. M., Centers, S. K. and Diovaldes, L. P. 1993. Cuban AIDS Policy. *The Lancet*, 342(8884), 1426.

Drazen, J. M., Kanapathipillai, R., Campion, E. W., Rubin, E. J., Hammer, S. M., Morrissey, S. and Baden, L. R.. 2014. Ebola and quarantine. *The New England Journal of Public Health*, 371, 2029–2030.

Eba, P. M. 2014. Ebola and human rights in West Africa. *The Lancet*, 384, 2091–2093.

Emrick, P., Christine, G. and Morowit, L. 2016. Ebola virus disease: international perspective on enhanced health surveillance, disposition of the dead, and their effect on isolation and quarantine practices. *Disaster and Military Medicine*, 2(13).

Encyclopaedia of Bioethics. 2004. New York: Macmillan.

Fidler, D. P. 1999. *International Law and Infectious Diseases*. Oxford: Clarendon.

Fidler, D. P. 2000. *International Law and Public Health: Materials on and Analysis of Global Health Jurisprudence*. Ardsley, NJ: Transnational.

Fidler, D. P. 2004. *SARS, Governance and the Globalization of Disease*. London: Palgrave Macmillan.

Fidler, D. P., Gostin, L. O. and Markel, H. 2007. Through the quarantine looking glass: drug-resistant tuberculosis and public health governance, law, and ethics. *The Journal of Law, Medicine and Ethics*, 35(4), 616–628.

Ford, N. L. and Quam, M. D. 1987. AIDS quarantine: the legal and practical implications. *The Journal of Legal Medicine*, 8, 353–397.

Forster, T. 1832. *Facts and Enquiries Respecting the Source of Epidemia*. London: Keating and Brown.

Fox, D. M. 1986. From TB to AIDS: value conflicts in reporting disease. *The Hastings Center Report*, 16(6), 11–16.

Gensini, G. F., Yacoub, M. H. and Contia, A. A. 2004. The concept of quarantine in history: from plague to SARS. *Journal of Infection*, 49, 257–261.

Gostin, L. O. 2000. *Public Health Law: Power, Duty, Restraint*. Berkeley, CA, Los Angeles, CA, and London: University of California Press.

Gostin, L. O. 2001. Public health, ethics and human rights: a tribute to the late Jonathan Mann. *Journal of Law, Medicine & Ethics*, 29(1), 121–130.

Gostin, L. O. and Curran, W. J. 1986. The limits of compulsion in controlling AIDS. *The Hastings Center Report*, 16(6), 24–29.

Gostin, L. O. and Lazzarini, Z. 1997. *Human Rights and Public Health in the AIDS Pandemic*. New York, NY: Oxford University Press.

Greene, J. T. 2015. Federal enforcement of mass involuntary quarantines: toward a specialized standing rules for the use of force. *Harvard National Security Journal*, 6, 58–111.

Gruskin, S. and Tarantola, D. 2002. Health and human rights. In Detels et al. (eds) *The Oxford Textbook of Public Health*, 4th edn (pp. 1–39). Oxford: Oxford University Press.

Hancock, T. 1821. *Researches into the Laws and Phenomena of Pestilence; Including a Medical Sketch and Review of the Plague of London in 1665; and Remarks on Quarantine*. London: W. Phillips.

Harris, A. and Martin, R. 2004. The exercise of public health powers in an era of human rights: the particular problems of tuberculosis. *Public Health*, 118(5), 313–322.

Heymann, D. L. 2014. Ebola: learn from the past. *Nature*, 514(7522), 299–300.

Hodge, J. G. Jr., Barraza, L., Measer, G. and Agrawal, A. 2014. Global emergency legal responses to the 2014 Ebola outbreak: public health and the law. *Journal of Law, Medicine & Ethics*, 42(4), 595–601.

Institute of Medicine. 1988. *The Future of Public Health*. Washington, DC: National Academic Press.

Jacobson v. Massachusetts, 197 U.S. 11, 25 S. Ct. 358, 49 L. Ed. 643 (1905).

Kamradt-Scott, A. Harman, S., Wenham, C. and Smith, F. III. 2015. *Saving Lives: The Civil-Military Response to the 2014 Ebola Outbreak in West Africa*. Sydney: University of Sydney. Available online at https://sydney.edu.au/arts/ciss/downloads/SavingLivesPDF.pdf (accessed November 16, 2016).

Khoshdel, A. R. 2014. Global war against Ebola and the role of military organizations. *Journal of Archives in Military Medicine*, 2(4), e25813.

Koch, T. 2015. Ebola, quarantine, and the scale of ethics. *Disaster Medicine and Public Health Preparedness*, 10(4), 654–661.

Koenig, K. L. 2015. Health care worker quarantine for Ebola: to eradicate the virus or alleviate fear? *Annals of Emergency Medicine. An International Journal*, 65(3), 330–331.

Kymlicka, W. 2002. Multiculturalism and minority rights: west and east: introductory essay. *Journal on Ethnopolitics and Minority Issues in Europe*, 4, 1–23.

Lane, J. D. and McNair, S. S. 2015. Sending soldiers to fight Ebola. *Military Medicine*, 180(6), 607–608.

Macklin, R. 1986. Predicting dangerousness and the public health response to AIDS. *Hastings Center Report*, 16(S6), 16–23.

Mann, J. M. (ed.). 1992. *AIDS and the World*. Cambridge: Harvard University Press.

Mann, J. M., Gostin, L., Gruskin, S., Brennan, T., Lazzarini, Z. and Fineberg, H. V. 1994. Health and human rights. *Health and Human Rights*, 1, 6–23.

Markel, H. 1997. *Quarantine!: East European Jewish Immigrants and the New York City Epidemics of 1892*. Baltimore, MD, and London: The Johns Hopkins University Press.

Markel, H. 2005. *When Germs Travel: Six Major Epidemics that Have Invaded America since 1900 and the Fears they Have Unleashed*. New York, NY: Pantheon.

McNeil, D. G. Jr. 2014. Using a tactic unseen in a century, countries cordon off Ebola-racked areas. *New York Times*. Available online at www.nytimes.com/2014/08/13/science/using-a-tactic-unseen-in-a-century-countries-cordon-off-ebola-racked-areas.html?_r=0 (accessed November 16, 2016).

Merritt, D. J. 1986a. The constitutional balance between health and liberty. *Hastings Center Report*, 16(6), 2–10.

Merritt, D. J. 1986b. Communicable disease and constitutional law: controlling AIDS. *New York University Law Review*, 61(5), 739–799.

National Academy of Sciences. 1986. *Confronting AIDS: Directions for Public Health, Health Care and Research*. National Academic of Sciences Study.

National Advisory Committee of SARS and Public Health. 2003. *Learning from SARS: Renewal of Public Health in Canada*. Ottawa: Health Canada. Available online at www.phac-aspc.gc.ca/publicat/sars-sras/pdf/sars-e.pdf (accessed December 8, 2016).

New York City Tuberculosis Working Group. 1992. Developing a system for tuberculosis prevention and care in New York City. In *The Tuberculosis Revival: Individual Rights and Societal Obligations in a Time of AIDS (Special Report Series)*. New York, NY: United Hospital Fund.

Novick, A. 1985. Quarantine and AIDS. *Connecticut Medicine*, 49(2), 81–83.

Parmet, W. E. 1985–1986. AIDS and quarantine: the revival of an archaic doctrine. law, social policy, and contagious disease: a symposium on Acquired Immune Deficiency Syndrome (AIDS). *Hofstra Law Review*, 14(1), 53–90.

Rothstein, M. A. 2015. Ebola, quarantine, and the law. *The Hastings Center Report*, 45(1), 5–6.

Rothstein, M. A., Alcalde, M. G., Elster, N. R., Majumder, M. A., Palmer, L. I., Stone, T. H. and Hoffman, R. E. 2003. *Quarantine and Isolation: Lessons Learned from SARS*. Louisville: Institute for Bioethics, Health Policy and Law, University of Louisville School of Medicine. Available online at www.iaclea.org/members/pdfs/SARS%20REPORT.Rothstein.pdf. (accessed December 8, 2016).

SARS Commission and Campbell, A. G. (eds). 2006. *The SARS Commission Final Report*. Ottawa: Ontario Ministry of Health and Long-Term Care.

Silva, D. S. and Smith, M. J. 2015. Limiting rights and freedoms in the context of Ebola and other public health emergencies: how the principle of reciprocity can enrich the application of the Siracusa Principles. *Health and Human Rights Journal*, 17(1), 52–57.

Stern, A. M. and Markel, H. 2004. International efforts to control infectious diseases, 1851 to present. *JAMA*, 292(12), 1474–1479.

Thompson, A. K. 2016. Bioethics meets Ebola: exploring the moral landscape. *British Medical Bulletin*, 117, 5–13.

Tomasevski K., Gruskin S., Lazzarini, Z. and Hendriks, A. 1992. AIDS and human rights. In J. M. Mann, D. Tarantola and T. Netter (eds) *AIDS in the World* (pp. 537–574). Cambridge, MA: Harvard University Press.

Towers, S., Patterson-Lomba, O. and Castillo-Chavez, C. 2014. Temporal variations in the effective reproduction number of the 2014 West Africa Ebola outbreak. *PLOS Currents Outbreaks*, 1.

UN Commission on Human Rights. 1984. The Siracusa Principles on the Limitation and Derogation Provisions in the International Covenant on Civil and Political Rights. 28 September 1984, E/CN.4/1985/4.

World Health Organization. 2000. Constitution of the World Health Organization (reprinted). *Bulletin of the World Health Organization*, 80, 983–984.

World Health Organization. 2006. Nonpharmaceutical interventions for pandemic flu. *Emerging Infectious Diseases*, 12(1), 81–87.

World Health Organization. 2015. *Successful Ebola Response in Nigeria, Senegal, and Mali*. Available online at www.who.int/csr/disease/ebola/one-year-report/nigeria/en (accessed November 16, 2016).

8 Ebola response and mandatory quarantine in the US military

An ethical analysis of the DoD "controlled monitoring" policy

Sheena M. Eagan

The United States in West Africa

In September 2014, President Obama committed up to 3,000 military service members to the Ebola response in West Africa. At this time, there were already a small amount of military advisors in West Africa. However, over the next several months thousands of US Department of Defense (DoD) service members deployed to this area, primarily Liberia. Their mission was mainly an engineering one: DoD teams built treatment centres, set up mobile testing labs, and provided transportation and logistical support. This support included planning, as well as the patching and preparation of airfields for the delivery of supplies (another major form of military response). Some service members also trained local health workers to use the newly built medical centres and laboratories. DoD service members were not involved in patient care or transport. In fact, DoD teams maintained contact primarily with other DoD personnel, stayed in DoD-approved lodging, ate DoD-approved food, and were monitored twice daily while deployed. These precautions were meant to minimize risk of exposure and infection.

Despite this population's low risk of exposure, US Defense Secretary Chuck Hagel announced the 21-day controlled monitoring policy in late October 2014. This policy applied to all US DoD service members returning from areas in West Africa affected by Ebola virus disease (EVD). Effectively a quarantine policy, the controlled monitoring program represented a significant departure from the national and international guidance regarding Ebola response and precautions. Expert opinion, the World Health Organization, and the US Centers for Disease Control were specific in not recommending mandatory quarantine and isolation. While the US DoD controlled monitoring policy drew little criticism or attention, civilian attempts to enforce mandatory quarantines were met with public critique and significant media scrutiny.

This chapter will analyze this policy and discuss the ethical issues involved. First, it will focus on the policy itself, examining the programmatic intent and motivation. After thoroughly examining the policy, this chapter will draw attention to the ethical issues involved in this new DoD policy. Ultimately it will argue that this policy poses serious ethical dilemmas as an unnecessary measure in disease control and as an excessive infringement on autonomy and individual rights. The chapter will also address ethical issues unique to the military context, specifically exploring the limited autonomy of enlisted and commissioned DoD service members.

The policy

On November 7, 2014, the Joint Chiefs of Staff released a detailed instruction outlining the new "controlled monitoring policy" for DoD personnel. This official instruction formalized a quarantine policy that was already being implemented by the Army (Montgomery, 2014). The official doctrine states:

> DoD service members, including active, reserve, and National Guard, will undergo a program of 21 days of controlled monitoring in a controlled monitoring area upon returning from deployment to, transitioning through, or having been stationed in the EVD outbreak area in West Africa as declared by the CDC.
>
> (Joint Chiefs of Staff, 2014a)

Importantly, although the decidedly softer term of "controlled monitoring" was used, this instruction detailed a program with all the components of a quarantine.[1] Officially, the terminology controlled monitoring was used to describe the program under which service members were "prohibited from having physical contact with family members and the general public" (Joint Chiefs of Staff, 2014a). Much like quarantine, controlled monitoring specifically restricted freedom of movement—limiting personal autonomy and liberty.[2] Although patients were not isolated individually, and were instead divided into cohorts (organized by time of entry and location), this asymptomatic, uninfected, and largely low-risk military population was still strictly segregated from the general population.

This policy represented a shift to a more "prudent" approach than the earlier policy of work-site, active-direct monitoring. The older policy enforced twice-daily active-direct monitoring for 21 days. Monitoring involved work-site interviews every day, including all nonduty days (weekend and off-days). In this policy, quarantine had only been recommended for those with "elevated exposure risk" (Joint Chiefs of Staff, 2014b). The earlier policy was similar to the recommendations put forth by the Centers for Disease Control (CDC) concerning EVD control.[3] Importantly, exemptions from the controlled monitoring program were granted to some populations. Those individuals and groups deemed to be "transient," primarily aircrews delivering supplies, were exempt from the mandatory controlled monitoring policy, as were all DoD civilian contractors. These populations were able to choose between controlled monitoring and workplace active-direct monitoring. Anyone entering controlled monitoring from this group did so voluntarily.

A "conservative and prudent response"

The US Department of Defense openly acknowledged that controlled monitoring represented a purposeful move towards a more "conservative and prudent" EVD response (Parrish, 2014). The Army released a series of statements explaining that this policy, which was supported by Army command and the Joint Chiefs, was part of a systematically cautious approach. Specifically, the 21-day quarantine was meant to protect not just those individual service members returning from West Africa but also their families, as well as the larger military and civilian communities to which they would return (Carroll and Harper, 2014). The novelty and public fear surrounding the disease also played into the decision, leading the DoD to be perhaps overly cautious, especially with the early cohorts of returning soldiers (Harper and Carroll, 2014).

These motives, denoting the prudence and cautiousness of the DoD policy, were reiterated throughout the military community and circulated throughout military-based press, such as *Stars and Stripes* (a newspaper available to service members on military bases at the Commissary or Exchange), base newsletters, command websites and military blogs. At the same time, information announcements circulated on the Armed Forces Network (AFN) radio and television, reassuring service members and their families that those deployed to EVD-affected areas were safe both in West Africa and when they returned. The press and public affairs offices also worked to reassure the military and surrounding civilian communities that they were taking all possible steps to ensure safety and avoid infection of others. These public information campaigns as well as the policy itself can be interpreted as an attempt to respond to or preempt a culture of fear within the military community, and American civilian community more generally. In fact, the Pentagon and military command cited discussion with service members and their families as one of the main motivations for the policy. There was a lot of fear surrounding the deployment of troops to EVD areas.

Civilian examples of mandatory quarantine

On the civilian side, forced mandatory quarantine for aid workers returning from EVD-affected areas was a highly contentious issue. Several states, including New York, New Jersey, Illinois, Georgia, and California, established policies involving mandatory quarantine (Denis, Sun, and Berman, 2014). These disease control measures were met with much debate, criticism, and media attention. Some believed that such measures were necessary, appealing to the same argument employed by the US DoD—prudent and cautious measures are necessary when dealing with a deadly infectious disease. These policies attempt to protect the public's health and welfare while assuaging the fear surrounding EVD. In fact, the North Carolina-based international relief group Samaritan's Purse, which had sent medical personnel to work in Liberia, instituted its own mandatory 21-day isolation for all returning staff members. The organization housed quarantined workers within a one-hour drive of medical facilities that were equipped to handle Ebola patients (such as the National Institutes of Health (NIH) or Emory University) (Denis, Sun, and Berman, 2014).

However, many other institutions, organizations, and groups did not agree with mandatory quarantine. The CDC, medical ethicists, public health experts, and even groups working on the front lines of the EVD outbreak were staunchly opposed to such mandatory requirements.[4] The US government's executive branch even weighed in, as the Obama administration laid out guidelines in response to these state-specific policies that called for voluntary isolation and monitoring of exposed individuals. Médecins Sans Frontières (MSF) argued that quarantine was neither warranted nor recommended (Park, 2014). Many public health experts pointed out that active monitoring is sufficient, owing to the fact that Ebola is not contagious until the presentation of symptoms, and others asserted that automatic mandatory quarantines could dissuade volunteers from providing aid to EVD-affected countries. Arguments surrounding the balance of personal freedom and public health were also highlighted in both the lay and academic press.

The level of attention and debate that civilian mandatory quarantine garnered provides an interesting juxtaposition to the DoD controlled monitoring policy. Discussion and critical examination were markedly absent with regard to the US DoD controlled monitoring policy; few articles mentioned this policy and there was little debate or commentary (Ackerman, 2014a). As well, while the aid workers involved in civilian cases of mandatory quarantine spoke out loudly, thousands of service members accepted mandatory quarantine in relative silence.

There are, of course, important differences between the mandatory quarantine of civilian aid workers and DoD service members. First, civilian aid workers represent a high-risk group, having provided care to EVD patients, while US DoD service members were not involved in patient care and thus were low (or no) risk. The difference in exposure warrants discussion of the DoD controlled monitoring program (Ackerman, 2014b). If the CDC, MSF, and American public were critical of mandatory quarantine for high-risk individuals such as returning aid workers—there should have been equal if not greater critique with regard to the mandatory quarantine of low-risk service members.

However, this lack of critique connects to the second important difference between these two populations: civilian aid workers enjoy a greater degree of autonomy and personal freedom than DoD service members. Service members represent a population with reduced autonomy who can be ordered to specific locations, including quarantine.[5] This fact undoubtedly contributed to the lack of critique on the part of the service members themselves, and likely also contributed to the lack of attention and protest from the American public. The normalcy of compulsory programs for service members was noted by President Barack Obama himself when discussing the controlled monitoring program. "we don't expect to have similar rules for our military as we do for civilians," Obama said. "[T]hey are already, by definition, if they're in the military under more circumscribed conditions" (Bradner, 2014). In the next section, this chapter will argue that the lack of autonomy and personal liberty within the military population represents an important consideration in ethical analysis. However, we will begin by examining the ethical dilemmas of mandatory quarantine more generally, before moving on to those dilemmas unique to a mandatory quarantine policy imposed on a military population.

Ethical issues

Public health policies, especially those dealing with infectious, epidemic diseases, are not without ethical dilemmas. Effective control of infectious disease often necessitates public health interventions that may reasonably infringe on the rights of individuals and limit their freedoms. Since infectious diseases, such as EVD, can be spread by an infected individual to others, it is understood to be unavoidable that public health may place restrictions or limitations on individuals in an attempt to protect the health of the larger population. In this way, public health interventions are rarely focused on the individual and instead are communitarian, contractarian, and utilitarian. However, the utilitarian paradigm and ability to impose public health interventions that infringe on individual rights is not unrestricted. Public health ethicists including Childress, Kass, and those involved in the Nuffield Council, among others, have proposed frameworks for ethical public health practice (Childress et al., 2002; Kass, 2001; The Nuffield Council on Bioethics, 2007). In fact, much discussion in this field has focused on the ethical issues associated with balancing individual rights and public protection in dealing with infectious diseases.[6]

In the case of liberty-limiting public health interventions, such as compulsory quarantine,[7] ethical justifications include a balance of the overall benefit to society, paternalism, and the classical harm principle.[8] As Phua argues, proponents of public health interventions, such as mandatory quarantine, often contend that these interventions can be justified by their overall benefits to society (Phua, 2013). Mandatory or forced public health interventions, and in fact public health interventions in general, often fall along the paternalistic spectrum, however when they specifically limit individual freedom the harm principle may be invoked.[9] Derived from the work of John Stuart Mill, the harm principle proposes that the only justification for interfering with an individual's liberty (against their will) is to prevent harm to others (Mill, 1869). The harm principle is highly relevant to public health, and has been used to specifically justify a variety of infectious disease control interventions including quarantine and isolation, as well as compulsory treatment.

When discussing the harm principle, and public health interventions that limit personal freedoms and liberty, it is important to consider other factors to insure ethically appropriate interventions. The Nuffield Council on Bioethics proposes the concept of a "liberty-limiting continuum" necessary to balance the harm principle, and thus for understanding when it is ethically permissible to restrict individual liberty and rights in an attempt to protect and promote community (population) health (The Nuffield Council on Bioethics, 2007). According to the Nuffield Council, quarantine has clear costs to individual liberty and ranks towards the top of the intervention ladder, or "liberty-limiting continuum" (The Nuffield Council on Bioethics, 2007). This classification is based on the grounds that quarantine restricts groups of individuals to specific locations, limiting their movement and activities. Moreover, quarantine is potentially the most costly to individual liberty as this program (which involves exposed but so far uninfected groups) restricts the freedom of more individuals, as opposed to isolation (which involves infected individuals). Quarantine also places uninfected individuals at risk of infection because they are possibly quarantined alongside infected people (The Nuffield Council on Bioethics, 2007). According to these ethical considerations, voluntary quarantine is the best option, and the most ethically acceptable. However, since mandatory quarantine may be permissible according to the harm principle and paternalistic understandings of public health, it is necessary to consider when and in what forms mandatory quarantine is an ethically permissible public health intervention.

According to Childress, a crucial component to the ethical permissibility of mandatory quarantine hinges on the effectiveness, necessity and proportionality of the intervention (Childress et al., 2002). Essentially, this type of restriction on personal liberty to benefit public health can only be justified if it is necessary, and will be an effective means of providing a proportional amount of benefit to the larger community.

Effectiveness: A program or policy that limits individual rights and liberties is not ethically justifiable unless it can be shown to be an effective means of disease control or health promotion (Childress et al., 2002; Kass, 2001). The DoD controlled monitoring program will not be officially evaluated, as the final program evaluation was delayed and later cancelled (Tilghman, 2014). That being said, there are ways in which this policy can be understood as effective. There were no cases of EVD within the controlled monitoring population, and no cases of EVD within the larger population upon reentry of the monitored groups. As well, the US DoD reported no complaints and no issues with the program. The lack of critique, and the withdrawal from West Africa (announced February 2015), served as the DoD's motivation to cancel the program evaluation. The programmatic intent and motivation for the controlled monitoring, as explicitly stated by military command, was the desire to be "prudent" and "conservative," taking into account larger, communitarian concerns of the military, dependents, and larger civilian population. On a macro level, quarantine has been historically effective in controlling epidemic disease, however its application in this low-risk population is perhaps a disproportionate response.

Proportionality and necessity: The condition of "proportionality" requires that the probable public health benefits are proportional to or exceed the harm done by limiting individual rights (Childress et al., 2002). According to Childress et al., positive features and good effects must be balanced against the negative features and effects of these interventions; the moral equation cannot be one-sided (Childress et al., 2002). While representing a decidedly prudent and cautious approach to disease control, the controlled monitoring policy constitutes a disproportionate response to EVD risks in its low-risk service member population. This population's personal freedom and liberty was restricted in explicit contradiction to CDC guidance for their exposure risk. The mere fact that a program will infringe on the rights and freedoms of individuals provides strong moral reason to look for alternatives that do not require this. The ethical practice of public health requires interventions that "minimize the infringement of general moral considerations" such as individual liberty even while basing decisions on larger utilitarian concerns (Childress et al., 2014). Identifying burdens and minimizing those burdens associated with public health interventions are ethically significant (Kass, 2001; Public Health Leadership Society, 2002). The controlled monitoring policy does not seek to minimize burdens on the individual, or to minimize infringement on individual liberty—instead opting for maximal infringement in attempt to insure health within the military community. As stated previously, this utilitarian or communitarian framework is common within public health but is not unrestricted.

In fact, it is this type of critique, on both ethical and scientific grounds, that led to widespread condemnation of mandatory quarantine policies for civilian aid workers returning to Illinois, New Jersey, and New York (Denis, Sun, and Berman, 2014; Park, 2014). In response to these policies, and the DoD controlled monitoring program, the CDC issued specific guidelines ruling out mandatory quarantines for people and populations who are asymptomatic (Carroll, 2014; CDC, 2014).

The limited autonomy of a military population

As mentioned earlier, there are relevant differences between the civilian cases being discussed and those military populations in "controlled monitoring." Specifically, the risk levels of these two populations warrant differing levels of disease precautions. However, there is another morally significant difference between these populations. As opposed to the civilian aid workers, DoD service members are a part of an institution that already limits their personal liberty and autonomy. The matter of limited autonomy represents an ethical issue unique to compulsory quarantine within the military context.

US Armed Forces service members were deployed to EVD-affected areas not by choice but by orders. Even if it is that case that some may volunteer for this particular mission, these women and men operate within an institutional and cultural environment of limited personal autonomy. The notion of following orders is foundational to the vertical cohesion that forms the military hierarchical structure and is understood as necessary for ensuring proper functioning. However, it means that one of the reasons that this population can be sent to mandatory quarantine (or controlled monitoring) is because military command has the ability to send them anywhere.

The concept of autonomy within the military, and the limited autonomy of the individual soldier, has been the subject of limited discussion within the ethical community, the most notable exception being research ethics, which has recognized the past abuse of this limited autonomy, often delineating military members as a vulnerable population. The limited autonomy and restricted personal liberty of the DoD service member is an important ethical consideration with regard to liberty-limiting public health interventions.

Within the military context, an individual service member hands over personal autonomy to the DoD upon enlistment or commission. Upon doing so, and becoming a member of the military profession they are expected to uphold and abide by the expectations of that profession. The military prioritizes the mission and expects loyalty and obedience from its service members (Eagan Chamberlin, 2014). Expectations of obedience and following orders are representative of the descriptive reality of the service member's life. The expectations related to obedience are clearly indicative of reduced autonomy. They are told where to live, where they can and cannot go, how to dress, and how to act. Owing to this limited autonomy, as well as the professional and institutional expectations of obedience, it should not be a surprise that service members and their families accepted mandatory controlled monitoring without critique. Following legal orders is essentially reflexive. Beyond that—as a service member there is also an expectation that policies and orders have been appropriately considered and evaluated at higher levels, eliminating the need for each individual to carefully analyze, evaluate, and consider its implications. The limited autonomy of service members, the expectations of obedience, and expectations of responsible decision-making at the command level forces questions regarding the responsibility of military command and the DoD to make appropriate policy decisions.

The stewardship model represents an excellent model for this responsibility, as it argues for the ethical use and not ownership of service members' autonomy. According to Block, "Stewardship is to hold something in trust[10] for another" (Block, 1993). Perhaps among the most significant contributions of the stewardship model to the military institution could be its conception of *use* as differentiated from *ownership*. As applied to the DoD, stewardship is specific in not granting ownership of whatever is being transferred—in this case the service member's autonomy—instead stewardship involves the right of use. Another key component of this concept is that according to the understanding of stewardship, the right to use the service member's autonomy is tempered. There is an obligation not to waste what one has been given a right to use. Instead there is an obligation to care for it (Block, 1993).

Service members have given up autonomy and personal liberty with the specific understanding that they will be used in the support of the military mission—for the protection and security of their nation. Although this expectation, and in fact this conception of the military mission, is normative and perhaps idealized, that does not negate the responsibilities of those parties entering into this agreement. Service members agree to a certain commitment of time, during which they forgo the autonomy to make choices normally granted to citizens and accept the explicit expectation of personal danger and self-sacrifice. Meanwhile, the military institution should have the obligation to use this power responsibly. The moral difference between ownership and use is foundational to the stewardship model—it is also a useful and powerful reminder in the military context that the lives of service members are not in fact owned by the DoD but rather available to them to use appropriately.

Essentially, a stewardship model has been in use on the battlefield for much of the history of organized warfare, although not specifically discussed in those terms. It is understood as impermissible for commanders to send those in their command forward without reason. The burden of command comes with a responsibility to care for the lives and welfare of the men (and now women) in your charge. It is only permissible for the lives of service members to be risked when there is cause. To do otherwise would be wrong and worthy of condemnation from other service members and the institution as a whole. For this reason, much effort and study has focused on effective ways to wage war, and military command is expected to base troop movement on a combination of proven methods and reliable intelligence.

The understanding of the stewardship model and the inherent obligation of military command to its service members, however, should not and does not stop at the edges of the battlefield. The movement of service member populations should always be done with informed cause and reason. While the DoD has the ability to give orders and deploy or move troops at any time owing to their reduced autonomy and obedience, this should not be unrestricted. The stewardship model as applied to the military context is built on an understanding that the service member's autonomy has been given to the DoD and is available to be used responsibly—it is not owned to be used without cause or valid reason. Rather, the use of service member autonomy should always be tempered by reasoned cause.

The stewardship model is particularly useful in the military context owing to the vulnerability that reduced autonomy creates. As a population unable to make self-governing decisions and instead beholden to the virtues of obedience and loyalty, cases may occur where service members are treated differently from non-service members without cause. The case of controlled monitoring represents a problematic use of the reduced autonomy of service members. The differing treatment between civilians, civilian contractors, and uniformed DoD service members challenges concepts of justice and fair treatment—forcing important questions about the validity of treating these populations differently in this instance. The service member population is accustomed to being told where to go; this however does not make mandatory quarantine appropriate. All movement of service members should be done with cause, and reasoning. The descriptive reality of the service member's reduced autonomy and obedience may weigh into ethical analysis, but does not negate a need for ensuring that public health interventions are proportionate, effective, and necessary.

Conclusion

In conclusion, the controlled monitoring program can be argued to have met its programmatic intent of being a conservative approach to disease control, and perhaps seemed prudent in a culture of uncertainty, fear, and anxiety within the larger military and American communities. However, this policy raises important ethical questions worthy of critique and examination. Why was this program not critiqued and evaluated? Why was it not discussed in the same way that mandatory civilian quarantines were? Is it ethically permissible to treat service members and civilians differently in this context? And was this an ethically appropriate infringement on and use of the limited autonomy of military service members?

The DoD and military command should not institute restrictive public health policies unless they can be justified. It seems inappropriate to restrict the liberty of large service member populations, against the advice of recognized institutions or agencies, such as the CDC, and in contradiction to general public health knowledge. To use service members' autonomy in an ethically responsibly way, they must only invoke their right to use this population's autonomy with cause and reason.

Notes

1 Quarantine refers to restrictions on the activities of a healthy person or group of people suspected of having been exposed to an infectious disease and who therefore might go on to develop it (Public Health Leadership Society, 2002). Quarantine is different from isolation, which isolates infected patients from the uninfected, healthy population. While the DoD does not use this term, the service member population is being placed into a designated facility because of the possibility of having been exposed to EVD by way of travel in Ebola-affected countries. The "controlled monitoring sites" can be understood as quarantines because they restrict the activities and movements of healthy but possibly exposed individuals. During this time, their individual liberty is restricted and they are not permitted to leave or have contact with others (beyond their cohort or health care providers).

2 Worthy of note is that military physicians were specifically instructed not to use the word "quarantine" when discussing this program with their patients, or other service members, although they often did so within their smaller medical peer groups.

3 According to the CDC,

> Asymptomatic individuals in the high risk category should have direct active monitoring for 21 days after the last potential exposure...have restricted movement within the community, and not travel on any public conveyances. Non-congregate public activities while maintaining a 3-foot distance from others may be permitted.
>
> (CDC, 2014)

Since these service members were not high-risk, the CDC recommended that they be "actively monitored until 21 days after the last potential exposure.... Individuals in this category do not require separation from others or restriction of movement within the community" (CDC, 2014).

4 While the Centers for Disease Control recommended some restrictions for high-risk individuals (such as those with direct exposure to the EVD patients), they have specifically not recommended mandatory quarantine. Although the CDC does not have jurisdiction or control over either individual states or the DoD, this does not negate the value of the guidance this agency provides. The CDC mission is founded on an understanding that it is, in fact, the "nation's health protection agency" (CDC, 2014).

5 For more on this topic, see section titled "The limited autonomy of a military population."

6 While there is no single framework for public health ethics, common threads emerge from the variety of frameworks currently discussed. Many frameworks for ethical public health intervention find their foundation in utilitarianism and communitarianism, however the individual remains an ethical consideration. As argued by the cited authors, ethical public health interventions strive to balance the protection of the public's health with individual rights. While individual rights may be superseded by larger utilitarian considerations, there are limits.

7 Although the current DoD policy does not explicitly use the term "quarantine," ethical analysis will analyze the policy as such, based on explanation given in endnote 1.

8 Voluntary quarantine is not being discussed here. When an individual voluntarily enters quarantine, or isolation for that matter, this changes the ethical context. Consenting to quarantine is the moral ideal and minimizes harm to individual liberty while protecting the public's health.

9 Since quarantine seeks to prevent harm to others by limiting the spread of disease, these interventions can be justified using the harm principle. However, the harm principle is not a single framework for public health ethics. Rather, the use of the harm principle illustrates that liberty-limiting interventions may be acceptable in order to prevent harm to others within the larger population (The Nuffield Council on Bioethics, 2007).

10 Importantly, although the term "trust" is used, stewardship is not specifically tied to the legal concept of trust and trusteeship, and should be understood as different.

References

Ackerman, S. 2014a. Conflicting Ebola guidelines puts US Defense Secretary in a tough spot. *Guardian.* Available online at www.theguardian.com/us-news/2014/oct/28/conflicting-ebola-guidelines-defense-secretary (accessed December 1, 2014).

Ackerman, S. 2014b. US troops on Ebola duty in Africa to face 21-day quarantine despite low risk. *Guardian.* Available online at www.theguardian.com/us-news/2014/oct/29/us-troops-ebola-face-21-day-quarantine-low-risk (accessed December 1, 2014).

Block, P. 1993. *Stewardship: Choosing Service over Self-interest.* San Francisco, CA: Berrett-Koehler.

Bradner, Eric. 2014. *Obama OK with Different Quarantine Policies for Military, Health Workers.* CNN.com Available online at www.cnn.com/2014/10/28/politics/obama-ebola-quarantine-disparity (accessed December 29, 2014).

Carroll, C. 2014. *Ebola Quarantine Optional for DOD Civilians.* Stripes.com. Available online at www.stripes.com/news/ebola-quarantine-made-optional-for-dod-civilians-1.311511 (accessed December 12, 2014).

Carroll, C. and Harper, J. 2014. *Hagel Approves 21-day Ebola Quarantine for Troops Returning from W. Africa.* Stripes.com. Available online at www.stripes.com/news/us/hagel-approves-21-day-ebola-quarantine-for-troops-returning-from-w-africa-1.311039 (accessed December 12, 2014).

Centers for Disease Control and Prevention. 2014. *Interim U.S. Guidance for Monitoring and Movement of Persons with Potential Ebola Virus Exposure (December 24 Update).* Available online at www.cdc.gov/vhf/ebola/exposure/monitoring-and-movement-of-persons-with-exposure.html (accessed December 29, 2014).

Childress, J. E; Faden, R. R., Gaare, R. D., Gostin, L. O., Kahn, J., Bonnie, R. J., Kass, N. E., Mastroianni, A. C., Moreno, J. D. and Nieburg, P. 2002. Public health ethics: mapping the terrain. *Journal of Law, Medicine & Ethics,* 30 (2002), 170–178.

Dennis, B., Sun, L. H. and Berman, M. 2014. N.Y., N.J., Illinois to impose new Ebola quarantine rules. *Washington Post.* Available online at www.washingtonpost.com/

national/health-science/ny-nj-governors-impose-new-ebola-quarantine-rules/2014/10/24/8096e43e-5bac-11e4-8264-deed989ae9a2_story.html (accessed December 29, 2014).

Eagan Chamberlin, S. 2014. The warrior in a white coat: moral dilemmas, the physician-soldier & the problem of dual loyalty. *Medical Corps International Forum*, 4, 4–7.

Harper, J. and Carroll, C. 2014. *Army Orders Soldiers into Isolation after Returning from Ebola Mission*. Stripes.com. Available online at www.stripes.com/army-orders-soldiers-into-isolation-after-returning-from-ebola-mission-1.310743 (accessed December 29, 2014).

Harper, J. and Carroll, C. *Joint Chiefs Recommend Quarantine for All US Troops Returning from West Africa*. Stripes.com. Available online at www.stripes.com/news/joint-chiefs-recommend-quarantine-for-all-us-troops-returning-from-west-africa-1.310929 (accessed December 1, 2014).

Joint Chiefs of Staff. 2014a. *Instruction Post Deployment, Policy for 21-Day Controlled Monitoring of DoD Service Members, Civilians, and Contractors Returning from Ebola Virus Disease Outbreak Areas in West Africa and CONUS*. Available online at www.defense.gov/home/features/2014/1014_ebola/docs/CJCSI%2042-0.01-Controlled-Monitoring-7-Nov-2014.pdf (accessed December 1, 2014).

Joint Chiefs of Staff. 2014b. *Pre-Deployment, Deployment and Post- Deployment Training, Screening and Monitoring Guidance for Department of Defense Personnel Deployed to Ebola Outbreak Areas*.

Kass, N. E. 2001. An ethics framework for public health. *American Journal of Public Health*, 91(11), 1776–1782.

Mill, J. S. 1869. *On Liberty*. London: Longman, Roberts & Green, 1869; Available online at www.bartleby.com/130 (accessed January 14, 2015).

Montgomery, N. 2014. *Quarantined General: Army Brass Unexpectedly Ordered Isolation of Soldiers Returning from Liberia*. Stripes.com. Available online at www.stripes.com/news/quarantined-general-army-brass-unexpectedly-ordered-isolation-of-soldiers-returning-from-liberia-1.310895 (accessed December 1, 2014).

Nuffield Council on Bioethics. 2007. *Public Health: Ethical Issues*. Cambridge: Cambridge.

Park, A. 2014. *Ebola Quarantines "Not Grounded on Science," Say Leading Health Groups*. Time.com. Available online at http://time.com/3542069/ebola-quarantines-not-grounded-on-science-say-leading-health-groups (accessed December 29, 2014).

Parrish, K. 2014. *DoD Sets Policy for Troops Returning from Ebola Areas*. Available online at www.defense.gov/news/newsarticle.aspx?id=123594 (accessed December 1, 2014).

Public Health Leadership Society. 2002. *Principles of the Ethical Practice of Public Health Version 2.2*. Available online at http://phls.org/CMSuploads/Principles-of-the-Ethical-Practice-of-PH-Version-2.2-68496.pdf (accessed December 1, 2015).

Phua, K. 2013. Ethical dilemmas in protecting individual rights versus public protection in the case of infectious diseases. *Infectious Diseases: Research and Treatment*, 2013(6), 1–5.

Tilghman, A. 2014. *DoD Extends Review of Ebola Quarantine Policy*. Militarytimes.com. Available online at http://militari.ly/16zEx8F (accessed December 29, 2014).

9 On the duty to care during epidemics

Daniel Messelken

Introduction

One of the most intriguing ethical issues in the context of epidemics and communicable diseases is the question whether doctors have a duty to provide medical care to a sick person even if doing so may put their own health at stake. With regard to the topic of this volume, the issue can be extended to include the question whether military health care personnel can be said to have a similar duty to provide care even in distant countries on behalf of their government.

Epidemics are usually defined as a widespread occurrence of a disease that affects a disproportionately large number of individuals within a region at the same time.[1] Epidemics very often involve contagious diseases that put everybody at risk who is staying, living, or working in such a region (or, at least, close to infected persons). A common reaction to epidemics therefore has always been to flee. One could label such a behavior as active "voluntary isolation" and from the perspective of avoiding an infection it is a perfectly reasonable and probably advisable action. It could however be argued that running away is a less acceptable action when it comes to physicians; they are needed to help during epidemics and they are the ones who have the knowledge and are given the resources to provide medical relief. Nevertheless, cases of physicians who refused to treat infectious patients or to work in a contagious environment have been reported during all kinds of epidemics (e.g., plague, AIDS, SARS). Therefore, when discussing ethical issues of epidemics, one sooner or later is confronted with the idea of the so-called "duty to care" (DTC) of health care personnel (HCP)—sometimes also labeled the "duty to treat" (with some different implications). An early (and positive) account of such a DTC has been given by the 1847 Code of the American Medical Association. It states that:

> when pestilence prevails, it is their [physicians'] *duty to face the danger*, and to continue their labors for the alleviation of the suffering, *even at the jeopardy of their own lives.*
>
> (Quoted in Zuger and Miles, 1987, p. 1926, emphasis added)

In the context of the recent Ebola virus disease (EVD) outbreak in West Africa, the questions of the duty to care and its limits arose, and the prevalence of the question was underlined by the high number of health care personnel who were infected while carrying out their work.

In addition, it is exactly the scarcity of medical resources that is often a main problem and main reason why epidemics cannot be stopped. Thus, more doctors and HCP who (voluntarily or based on their duties) expose themselves to the risky work environment are often needed to stop an epidemic. The call from Médecins Sans Frontières (MSF), which was one of the first organizations to respond to the Ebola outbreak in 2014 and remained among the main actors to fight the epidemic, is a good illustration of this necessity. Its president, during a speech at the United Nations, urged:

> To curb the epidemic, it is imperative that *states* immediately deploy *civilian and military assets* with expertise in biohazard containment…. To put out this fire, we must run into the burning building.
> (Joanne Liu, quoted in Médecins Sans Frontières, 2015, p. 13, emphasis added)

The pure fact that MSF *publicly* called for support from *military* actors may serve as a proof of the urgency. But the metaphor of "running into the burning building" also gives us hints about the nature of the DTC. It suggests for example that it is not everybody's duty: we would not expect a normal bystander to run into a burning building but we would expect a fireman to do it. And then: if he is a fireman, can he refuse to enter the building because it is dangerous? Does he need to ask permission to run into the burning building? What kind of support can he expect to receive?

Coming back to the issue of a DTC of doctors, the main question has been formulated in a concise manner in the following way:

> Do physicians, nurses, and other healthcare workers have a duty to care for patients when doing so exposes the workers themselves to significant risks of harm and even death?
> (Malm et al., 2008, p. 4)

This question shall in this chapter be amended by a second layer: what are the possible role and obligations of military HCP in the context of epidemics? Do members of the military health care services (and their personnel) have a different DTC than their civilian counterparts?

Outline and aims of the chapter

First, we will look at the concept of the duty to care and apply or transfer the concept to the situation of an epidemic like the recent Ebola outbreak. As the most commonly discussed case in the literature is that of the DTC of doctors and

HCP for their patients within their society we will start with this reduced perspective. Later, we will widen the perspective in order to include international aspects and challenges of epidemics such as the situation that occurred in the context of the EVD outbreak. A final consideration will deal with the questions surrounding why and to what extent the DTC of military HCP may be different from that of their civilian counterparts. Thus, with this chapter, we aim on the one hand to give an overview of the existing literature on the duty to care; on the other hand, we want to provide ethical arguments on the justification of a duty to care and to analyze the scope and the limits of the DTC on several levels (national/international, civilian/military, norm/emergency).

The concept of a duty to care of physicians and other HCP

This first section of this chapter will be dedicated to an analysis of the idea of a "duty to care" (DTC), according to which physicians and other health care personnel (HCP) are morally obligated to treat people in need of medical assistance, *even if doing so puts the HCP at some risk*. These ideas and the ethical principles that will be found are relevant also for military health care personnel insofar as there is widespread agreement, that "[e]thical principles of health care do not change in times of armed conflict and other emergencies and are the same as the ethical principles of health care in times of peace" (International Committee of the Red Cross (ICRC) et al., 2015).

The general duty to rescue and a role-related duty to care

Before reviewing the arguments in favor and against a specific duty to care for HCP that can be found in the philosophical literature,[2] we will first provide some thoughts about a general duty to rescue. It is commonly agreed upon that everybody has a general duty to rescue others who are in need of help and if the rescuer can provide that support without too high costs for him or herself. This principle has been famously formulated by Singer, who also gave a common example for such a case:

> [I]f it is in our power to prevent something very bad from happening, without thereby sacrificing anything morally significant, we ought, morally, to do it. An application of this principle would be as follows: if I am walking past a shallow pond and see a child drowning in it, I ought to wade in and pull the child out. This will mean getting my clothes muddy, but this is insignificant, while the death of the child would presumably be a very bad thing.
>
> (Singer, 1972, p. 231)

Obviously, there would not be such a stringent duty if the child was not drowning in a small pond but in the open sea and if the rescuer was unable to swim. Thus, the prima facie duty to rescue can be qualified according to the circumstances and the skills of the rescuer. Capabilities and special competencies can, on the other hand, also justify a duty that goes beyond the general duty to help of everybody. We label such obligations *role-specific duties*, which Brody and Avery describe in the following way for the medical profession:

> All members of society have an ethical duty to rescue others in dire need of help when they are in a position to do so. Physicians arguably have a role specific duty of rescue by virtue of their medical competence to provide the help that victims of infectious outbreaks require.
>
> (Brody and Avery, 2009, p. 41)

This is not only a recent position in the literature but can be tracked back through history. In the context of epidemics, a professional duty is famously referred to by Boghurst, a seventeenth-century pharmacist who associated specific duties to professions in a commentary he wrote on the pestilence in Europe:

> Every man that undertakes to bee of a profession or takes up on him any office must take all parts of it, the good and the evill, the pleasure and the pain, the profit and the inconvenience altogether, and not pick and chuse; for ministers must preach, Captains must fight, Physitians attend upon the Sick, etc.
>
> (William Boghurst, 1666, as quoted in Zuger and Miles, 1987, p. 1925)

In this short quote, we find the argument that by choosing a profession one inevitably accepts the advantages and disadvantages that come with that profession. Maybe one chooses being a doctor because of the reputation that is usually associated with the profession, but then one also has to accept the typical obligations of that profession, namely to attend patients in need of medical care that may also constitute a danger for the physician.

But are such professional obligations unconditional? How far do professional duties go and how much danger can HCP be morally expected to accept in a situation like that of an epidemic? This is the question we want to shed some light on in the following section and that has been formulated by Malm and colleagues from a more modern perspective referring to role-related positive duties. They ask

> whether healthcare workers, in virtue of their role as healthcare workers, have a special positive duty to treat that obliges them to take greater risks in their efforts to aid others than would be required of persons in general.
>
> (Malm et al., 2008, p. 7)

The "standard case" discussed in the literature is usually restricted to a national level and we will restrict our literature review in the first section accordingly before widening the focus in the second section. In this context, the question of HCPs' duty to care was mostly discussed as a reaction to HIV in the 1980s and after the SARS epidemic in 2002/03. For the theoretical debate, the issue of possible bioterrorist attacks also played a minor role (see, e.g., Alexander and Wynia, 2003).

Arguments in favor of a professional DTC

Several arguments in favor of a professional DTC can be found in the literature. The different approaches can be labeled the choice model, the rights model, the social contract model, the consent model, the virtue model, and the capabilities model.

Individual physician–patient contract: the "choice model"

Probably the most obvious justification of the duty to care of physicians emerges out of the contract between a patient and the physician. If someone sees a doctor and the latter accepts him as a patient, then she also accepts the duty to care for that patient. This is what the patient is asking for and what the contract is all about. This model, however, does not provide an argument for a more general duty to care of doctors or health care personnel vis-à-vis members of society in general. Whereas doctors are, in normal circumstances, allowed to reject patients if there is no emergency, their acceptance of patients makes them enter the special physician-patient-relationship with its duties and obligations. As a result,

> Doctors and nurses owe a greater duty of beneficence to patients than the average person.... So, although there is arguably a duty of beneficence to both patients and non-patients, it is a more stringent requirement in the first group than in the second.
>
> (Sokol, 2003, p. 22)

We could label this first argument in favor of a DTC the "choice model" as it presupposes a choice of both the patient ("Which doctor am I going to?") and the physician ("Am I accepting this person as a patient?"). The DTC, in this model, is limited to an established physician–patient relationship based on an individual contract.

Individual right to health: the "rights model"

A second argument, on the basis of which a duty to care for physicians and health care personnel can be justified, is the individual (natural) right to health care that is also part of the Universal Declaration of Human Rights (Article 25). If everybody has a right to receive adequate health care, there must also be an obligation for someone to provide that care. Thus, according to the so-called rights model,

> a patient's right to health care creates a correlative duty on the part of physicians, institutions, or society to provide health care.
>
> (Zuger and Miles, 1987, p. 1926)

However, as the quote suggests, no direct obligation or direct duty for individual doctors can be deduced from the rights model. Thus, even if we assume an individual (natural or human) right to decent health care, it remains unclear who can be individually held responsible to provide it. Within the rights model, it is the state or society that has a duty to provide care and individual doctors usually do not have, within this approach, a direct obligation to provide medical care to everybody. As human rights bind states and not individuals, the rights model can only be used to justify indirect duties for certain groups of doctors—namely those also *employed* by the state as "immediate agents of society's duty to fulfill the right to medical care" (Zuger and Miles, 1987, p. 1927).

The reciprocity view: the "social contract model"

A third approach to justify physicians' obligation to treat all members of society and to accept some risk during the exercise of their profession is based on a social contract argument. Society invests considerable resources into the education of physicians and also grants the profession important privileges (monopoly, recognition, remuneration); in return, they expect that physicians provide society with the health care it needs—in normal but also in more difficult circumstances. Malm and colleagues label this the reciprocity view:

> The reciprocity view thus asserts that in exchange for all these benefits, healthcare workers have a duty to treat that can oblige them to incur a greater than normal risk to themselves.
>
> (Malm et al., 2008, p. 10)

We could talk of an implicit social contract as the argument is seldom spelled out as above even though the investment into medicine by the state certainly is based on the expectation that a decent health care provision will be achieved. Wynia describes the relationship between the partners to the social contract as one of trust:

> We believe the most compelling reason for a duty to treat stems from medicine's social contract and its trustee relationship with the public.... This requires that the profession provide care not only in times of good health, but more importantly, in times of ill health.
>
> (Wynia et al., 2006, p. 152)

In a similar way than in the quote of Boghurst above, we can find that by accepting the positive sides of a profession one has to accept its downsides, too. In the case of medicine, we can add the fact that physicians are usually granted a monopoly, which adds to the social trust:

> Just as the police have a duty to protect defenseless citizens based on their monopoly over the legitimate use of force, so physicians have a duty to treat those in medical need, even in the face of some personal risk.
>
> (Arras, 1988, p. 11)

The question then remains what "some personal risk" could mean and, accordingly, what level of risk has to be accepted as part of the social contract.

Consent to some level of risk by choosing the profession:
the "consent model"

A fourth argument in favor of a DTC explicitly takes into account the risk-taking that a DTC would entail under circumstances like epidemics. Against the possible assertion that such risk could reduce the persuasiveness of a DTC of health care personnel, it has been argued that

> Like other public service professions, including the fire and police forces, some risk is simply part of the job description for medical professionals.
>
> (Huber and Wynia, 2004, p. W10)

The statement that "risk is part of the job" can certainly be subscribed to by many (or even all) physicians. Treating patients always includes some aspects of risk as they may have communicable diseases without even knowing it. In addition, the clinical environment brings together patients with different kinds of diseases. As this is clear from the beginning, health care personnel know about the risks associated with their jobs and do agree to share it. Daniels formulates this point in the following way with an important qualification:

> The general mechanism for distributing the benefits and burdens of risk-taking is, and should be, consent. Consequently, if physicians have a duty or obligation to take certain risks, it must be the result of their agreeing to do so.
>
> (Daniels, 1991, p. 38)

This leaves us with two issues. First, consent to such kind of risk should be given explicitly and may for example be part of the job description when starting a new position. Second, the question remains what kind of risk can HCP be expected to accept without an explicit consent or in situations when the risk cannot be exactly described—as may be the case during the outbreak of an epidemic. In those cases, we cannot base our argument on what may be labeled a normal risk level (accepted by becoming physicians) and thus would need a different approach. The acceptable risk level would need to be based on what can be reasonably expected and for example also be balanced against competing claims (like the protection of the HCPs' families). The acceptable risk level may also be related to the specialty of a doctor: an epidemiologist has to agree to a different acceptable risk level than an ophthalmologist.

Virtuous physician: the "virtue model"

A related argument can be found in the virtue model, according to which caring for patients and the acceptance of some risk during doing so are among the characters of the good physician (see Zuger and Miles, 1987, p. 1927).

However, the virtue account is also not without preconditions. Most importantly, it "depends upon a historically grounded and voluntarily sustained commitment to a particular notion of the good physician as someone who takes risks for a patient" (Arras, 1988, p. 15). As such a commitment is neither historically proven nor uncontroversial today, the virtue model seems to stand on a rather weak basis. Nevertheless, one important advantage of the virtue account would be that it could justify duties for *individual* doctors and not "only" the profession as such. As Arras puts it,

> A virtue-based duty to treat has to condemn voluntaristic arrangements as systematic evasions of individual duty.... Those who refuse to treat are bad physicians, even if they succeeded in referring all of their would-be patients to other doctors.
>
> (Arras, 1988, p. 15)

Special training: the "capabilities model"

A final argument on why doctors and HCP have a more stringent DTC for infected persons than normal people have can be found in the special training they have received. On the one hand, this argument shares similarities with the social contract and consent model as capabilities are associated with duties. On the other hand, the capabilities model also has a consequentialist aspect insofar as

> given that healthcare professionals know how to aid others, they can provide that aid more efficiently, perhaps by doing more with fewer resources or doing more in less time, than nonprofessionals can.
>
> (Malm et al., 2008, p. 9)

Someone who is better trained to deliver aid accordingly has a stronger obligation to do so. Prima facie, this argument is convincing and we have seen a similar rationale when introducing the duty to rescue. It can, however, also lead to counterintuitive consequences as it may discourage people from striving for capabilities like treating infectious diseases if such skills later create a (too strong) moral obligation to risk one's life.[3] Therefore, duties that are directly associated to special capabilities should be balanced in order not to prevent people from striving for knowledge.

Individual physicians' versus the medical profession's DTC

A DTC can thus be stipulated in different ways by the different approaches and models presented in the above section. An important distinction has to be amended with regard to the addressee of a duty to care, which can either be an individual physician or the medical profession as a whole (see Zuger and Miles, 1987, p. 1927), depending on the justification model referred to.

Most obviously, the choice model creates a positive duty of an individual physician to care for an individual patient when a physician–patient relationship based on a contract already exists. In a less direct way, *individual* physicians are also bound by the virtue and capabilities models depending on their perception of the physicians' role and the capabilities they have. On the other hand, most of the approaches discussed above address the medical profession as a whole, without stipulating an individual duty to care. This can be said for the rights, social contract, consent, virtue, and capabilities models. Based on these approaches, one can argue in favor of a general DTC of the members of the medical profession, without however justifying a DTC of an individual physician as long as others would be in a position to equally take over the obligation.

Arguments against the DTC

In contrast to the arguments favoring a DTC of physicians vis-à-vis patients, the philosophical literature also offers counterarguments or at least arguments for a restriction of such a duty.

Conflicting obligations: which role supersedes the others?

A first and important argument that qualifies the DTC concedes that doctors do not only have obligations stemming from their role as doctor but, like all people, have different obligations stemming from their different roles. Thus, the concept of the DTC can be criticized as it

> fails to consider the holder of the duty as a multiple agent belonging to a broader community. Doctors, in such situations, play several incompatible roles—doctor, spouse, parent, for example—and they must deal with them as best they can. The limits of the duty of care are thus also defined by the strengths of competing rights and duties.
>
> (Sokol, 2006, p. 1239)

This means that, however stringent and far-reaching the obligations from the medical role with respect to a DTC might be, these duties need to be balanced against competing duties before we can state the extent of the DTC in any concrete situation. During epidemics and other situations, which involve a certain risk during the exercise of medical care, the DTC may thus be limited and doctors may rightfully invoke the limits of their medical duties. According to Sokol,

> The current patient-centered climate has obscured the rights of healthcare professionals, often reducing them to mere service providers.... A person's right to treatment does not trump another person's right to self-preservation.
>
> (Sokol, 2003, pp. 24f.)

Thus, even though the doctor role might impose a prima facie DTC on physicians, they could well claim that obligations associated to other roles or just oneself reduce the authority and scope of the DTC.

DTC must be weighed against risk

Obviously, no one can reasonably be expected to take any risk to help others, whatever the risk may be. This is true with regard to the general duty to rescue and the same argument also sets limits to the DTC of doctors. In the end, it is about finding an agreement on what level of risk HCP can be expected to accept because of their role as HCP.[4] Arras summarizes this problem in a convincing manner:

> The most that can be said here, I think is that gauging the precise threshold between strict duty and supererogation will always be a matter of practical judgment strongly influenced by socially and historically determined views of what counts as a "reasonable risk". Procedurally, this requires an ongoing dialogue between professionals on the firing line and the rest of society.
>
> (Arras, 1988, p. 16)

There is, however, also a second line of argument why HCP should not be expected to accept any risk to their own health and survival. According to this position, the DTC

> should be attenuated, but not eliminated, by the physician's responsibility not to become a patient him or herself. Risks must be balanced against one's own capacity to do good in the future, and while heroism is to be commended, martyrdom is not often called for.
>
> (Huber and Wynia, 2004, p. W9)

Even though it would be more convincing to weigh against the probability of someone's future doing good, this consequentialist argument has an important point. Especially during epidemics, HCP are themselves a "scarce resource" and they can only help in the fight against an epidemic as long as they are not infected themselves. Thus, heroic risk-taking does not make sense from an overall perspective but rather well reflected acceptance of a limited and circumscribed risk.[5]

Effectiveness of the treatment

Along a similar line of argument, the effectiveness of available treatments may also limit the DTC. This position is put forward by Sokol:

> If, however, the lack of protective equipment means that the chances of infection are high and no, or trivially small, benefits will result for the

patients (as is often the case with Ebola), then the doctor may justifiably abandon the doomed patients.

(Sokol, 2006, p. 1240)

According to his argument, "virtuous patients" (ibid.) would not expect doctors and health care personnel to run too much of a personal risk in order to care for rather hopeless patients in desperate circumstances and given the unavailability of effective treatment.

Hence, as for the care of "normal" diseases during "normal" times, the possibility of a cure is a precondition to a duty to care—and even more when the latter is associated with an important level of risk for the care-provider. Caring for seemingly hopeless patients without a proven cure would still be a praiseworthy action, but may well be supererogatory and thus beyond a duty to care.

Section summary: scope and limits of the DTC

Contrary to the viewpoint that a duty to care has no "convincing basis" (Malm et al., 2008, p. 16) or could only be based on an "elusive" argument (Brody and Avery, 2009, p. 46) and thus "is too vague to be helpful" (Sokol, 2006, p. 1240), we have shown that a DTC can rely on different arguments. Thus, according to our analysis, a DTC of doctors and HCPs exists and may also include an obligation to take some risks. It can be justified in a general manner by the duty to rescue and then be extended through the different more specific arguments that consider the role-related obligations of the medical professions. The scope and the limits of the DTC of doctors and HCP are however not always clearly defined and would need further attention. The latter was also one of the conclusions of a board of experts who reviewed the question after the SARS outbreak in Canada:

> We could not reach consensus on the issue of duty to care, particularly regarding the extent to which healthcare workers are obligated to risk their lives in delivering clinical care.
>
> (Singer et al., 2003, p. 1343)

Thus, we have to accord that the limits of the DTC do depend on contextual factors and need to be negotiated and defined. The circumstances do however not alter the general ethical principles, as has been agreed upon recently by a number of important organizations:

> 1. Ethical principles of health care do not change in times of armed conflict and other emergencies and are the same as the ethical principles of health care in times of peace.
>
> (International Committee of the Red Cross (ICRC) et al., 2015)

Thus, as much as difficult circumstances like emergencies influence the application of ethical principles and add a layer of complexity to the contextual factors, the underlying arguments remain unchanged.[6]

An internationalized DTC: "run into the burning building"

The review of the academic literature in the first section of this chapter revealed that arguments in favor of a duty to care can be based on a variety of justifications. None of the arguments presented justifies however an unconditional DTC or comes without preconditions. The questions of the extent of the DTC and its addressee emerged as the main points of contention and they become even more complex during international health crisis when international actors come into play. This is for example the case when humanitarian actors or military personnel (including HCPs) are sent abroad on humanitarian missions to "fight" epidemics like Ebola. As the existing literature considers largely a civilian context and is focused strongly on the national level, it seems necessary and interesting to widen the horizon in order to analyze the duty to care on several levels and to leave the level of the physician–patient relationship within a given society. The following section presents arguments in favor of a broader understanding of the concept of the "duty to care" as a state-centered duty on the one hand but also to explain how this expanded duty to care may justify the imposition of risks on "state doctors"—doctors and HCPs who are employed by the state and therefore have a special obligation vis-à-vis the state and to implement the state's policy.

Arguments in favor of a state-centered DTC (collective, international)

The term DTC has usually been used to refer to a duty of a physician vis-à-vis a patient or a sick person more generally. During (international) epidemics, this relationship can however not describe all relevant aspects and the following section shall therefore elaborate on a state-centered duty to care for the victims of an epidemic.

Containment of the epidemic

A first group of arguments, according to which states can be ascribed a moral duty to react to the outbreak of epidemics, can be constructed around the aim of containing the spread of an epidemic.

A. Egocentric, selfish argument: In a rather selfish way, states have an interest to contain the outbreak of epidemics even abroad and outside their own territory, in order to limit the spread to the states or region where the epidemic emerged and to prevent expansion to other parts of the world. One can describe a state's reaction aiming at the containment of an epidemic abroad as self-defense in the sense that the state tries to avert the threat of the epidemic to its own citizens (see Gilbert's contribution to this volume). Such an argument however overlooks the fact that an epidemic cannot be attributed to an attacker against whom the act of self-defense could be directed. Also, arguments of self-defense are usually invoked to justify (violent) actions that would not be (morally) allowed without the context of self-defense. Actions that aim at containing an epidemic in most cases however would not need this extra level of justification even though they may be costly. A more convincing argument why states may have an interest to intervene against epidemics outside their own territory seems to be the simple consequentialist calculus that harm can be reduced by containing the spread of an epidemic disease.

B. Public health argument: Actions to assist countries and people in need of medical aid to stop an epidemic can often be morally justified on the basis of public health ethics and do not require a reference to self-defense. Typical measures and actions within the public health framework would for example include isolation and/or quarantine of infected people or suspect cases, and travel restrictions to and from risk areas. Similarly, the (maybe simplified or less restrictive) use of experimental drugs and the compassionate use of existing treatment can be justified by public health ethics. Less obviously, the use of resources both at home and abroad, including sending missions of experts to affected areas, may fall under public health measures if they constitute a necessary or at least promising means to protect a state's own population.

Principle of humanity: solidarity and compassion

Another moral argument upon which a state-centered DTC can rely is the principle of humanity. It is the fundamental principle of international humanitarian law and thus regulates the relations between states during conflict, but the principle explicitly also refers to the protection of health as one of the purposes of humanitarian action. According to the ICRC doctrine, the principle of humanity demands

> to prevent and alleviate human suffering wherever it may be found. Its purpose is to protect life and health and to ensure respect for the human being.[7]

By intervening in Ebola-affected regions (or during other epidemics), states can clearly act according to the principle of humanity and show their solidarity with those who are suffering. Thus, the principle can provide a reason why (medical) intervention is justified and may, if the principle is taken to be more demanding, also provide the basis for a more stringent duty to assist. As epidemics in addition often happen to affect the poorer regions of the world, where medical systems have fewer capacities, the aspect of solidarity may be brought into play as a reaction to these inequalities. Dawson takes the following stance in the context of the recent EVD outbreak:

> I think it's important to see this Ebola outbreak against the background of global injustice in relation to health.
>
> (Dawson, 2015, p. 109)

It remains open, however, to what extent the general principle of humanity or arguments based on solidarity can eventually justify a state-centered DTC during epidemics or whether they instead describe paths of actions that are clearly praiseworthy but remain supererogatory nevertheless.[8]

An analogy to the Responsibility to Protect (R2P)

A last argument to provide a state-centered DTC that I want to briefly elaborate on is based on the so-called "Responsibility to Protect" (International Commission on Intervention and State Sovereignty et al., 2001). According to this paradigm, states have a responsibility to protect their populations from serious harm, namely from man-made violence like war, genocide, or ethnic cleansing. This responsibility is primarily one of each state on their own territory, but can become an international one if states are not able or are unwilling to fulfill it and act accordingly domestically.

Beyond the mentioned cases of man-made violence, the Responsibility to Protect also extends to natural disasters. In the original report on R2P, one can find as a possible trigger of such state responsibility the existence of:

> overwhelming natural or environmental catastrophes, where the state concerned is either unwilling or unable to cope, or call for assistance, and significant loss of life is occurring or threatened.
>
> (International Commission on Intervention and State Sovereignty. et al., 2001, p. 33)

I would suggest that epidemics like the 2014–15 EVD outbreak clearly meet these criteria as the consequences of the outbreak were both overwhelming for the local health care system and came with (or threatened to cause) a significant loss of life. Accordingly, epidemics on a comparable scale can trigger the state responsibility to protect on several levels (from local to international) and during different phases of their occurrence (prevention, acute and long-term reaction). As adequate reactions to an epidemic threat will consist of the provision of medical care and other public health measures, one can well argue that an R2P reaction to the natural catastrophe of an epidemic creates a state-centered DTC, first domestically and if that is not sufficient also on an international level.

Section summary: a broader and different understanding of the DTC

The arguments for a state-centered DTC, developed in the subsections above, all have in common that 1) the resulting duties of states would be broader than those of individual doctors and 2) that state-centered duties or responsibilities are based on a different logic than the DTC of individual doctors that was argued for in the first section of this chapter.

Special role and role-related DTC of military HCPs

One of the points that arose out of the discussion of the DTC earlier in this chapter was that the resulting duty during epidemics would rather be a state-centered duty. As a result, it then addresses state doctors and HCPs or the medical profession as a whole rather than individual doctors. One group of "state doctors" is composed of those physicians who are employed by and serve in the armed forces: military doctors. Military doctors may play a prominent role in combatting epidemics and may have a special duty to do so for several reasons that we want to look at in this section.

Role-related argument

A theoretical argument that brings into play the military medical services and may ethically justify their deployment (domestically or abroad) can be developed under the assumption that there is, during epidemics, a state-centered DTC or duty to assist. As we have already briefly discussed above, military doctors and HCPs can, like emergency doctors and those working in public hospitals, be interpreted as being part of those state doctors who are "immediate agents of society's duty to fulfill the right to medical care" (Zuger and Miles, 1987, p. 1927). As a result of being part of that group, their duty to care for *all* sick persons is stronger than that of private physicians. In addition, the question of which persons fall under "all sick persons" can in the case of state doctors be answered as those sick individuals whom the state has a duty to care for. Obviously, this covers first and foremost its own population; but under the provisions of the Responsibility to Protect or the principle of humanity this group can be understood in a more extensive manner. The scope of the DTC for state doctors is then much larger than it is for private physicians, and the limitations of the DTC, e.g., by risks, are less clear and may be far more demanding.

One could object that the task of military HCPs consists of and is limited to caring for their comrades (and, during armed conflict, for the sick and wounded persons independent of their affiliation). Yet, similar arguments could be brought forward to restrict the tasks and possible deployment of other military personnel to strict cases of a state's self-defense. Nevertheless, they are sent into humanitarian missions without a clear link to their countries' self-defense from time to time and cannot refuse to participate. In a similar way, and for example in connection with R2P arguments or under the principle of humanity, states can justify the deployment of adequate means to counter health crises—with medical support missions being one of these means. In the end, it is therefore a political decision whether an "Ebola deployment" or similar missions are part of the job description of military doctors even if such kind of deployment has not much been envisaged only some years ago. As however some insecurity about the nature and location of deployments is also part of their job, military HCP probably have to accept changes to their tasks and the forms of deployment they are sent to.

If arguments on a state-centered DTC became increasingly accepted, a discussion about the possible missions of military medical services should likewise be initiated. A similar debate was briefly engaged in late 2014 under the heading of "White Helmet Troops," an international rapid-response unit tasked to deal with epidemic outbreaks.[9] The role of being a military doctor could, as a result of such a development, in the future clearly include the obligation to work in missions sent to fight epidemics.

Capabilities-related argument

Another rather pragmatic argument in favor of the deployment of military HCP during epidemics refers to their special skills. They have the knowledge (e.g., from biological warfare training), the funding, and the necessary resources and logistics to quickly set up missions that can effectively succeed in combatting epidemic outbreaks. They simply can do the job; and then it is not only the case that "ought implies can" but sometimes also "can implies ought." This argument is, in the end, a typical example of a role-related DTC as described in the capabilities model presented earlier.

Limitations by risk

If we follow the arguments above, military HCPs have a "transitive" DTC as state agents, which they inherit from the state that is the virtual addressee of the duty. Like a direct DTC, the transitive duty is however neither unconditional nor without limitations and has to take into account the risk that is imposed upon the person who is ordered to fulfill the duty. In our context, this would be the military medical personnel. Even though danger is part of the military job description and military medical personnel are more willing to accept risks than their civilian counterparts, the imposition of risks must nevertheless be weighed and justified. The risks associated with the work required during epidemics like an EVD outbreak are not the ones commonly encountered on military service. One would rather expect that risks associated with conflict and fighting have to be accepted by military HCP. The risks that come with a humanitarian deployment into a region with an epidemic may be on a similar level but are of a very different kind. The military HCP may thus claim not to be prepared to face these risks if they did not or do not receive an adequate training and the necessary resources.

We can therefore conclude that there are valid arguments why military HCP may have an inherited DTC that extends even to risky missions abroad. Such conclusions however also call for a careful revision of the role, ethical obligations, and typical deployment scenarios of military health care personnel in order to avoid misconceptions.

Open issues

Before concluding this chapter, we would like to briefly mention some open issues that are associated with the concept of a duty to care during epidemics and that could not be discussed with the attention they would merit.

Epistemic uncertainty of the risk

As we have seen, one of the central determinants of the scope of the DTC is the level of risk associated with the task of providing (medical) care for an infectious person. This raises the epistemic problem that the definition of a "risk" is always and notoriously vague. This makes the already difficult task of weighing the different obligations of HCP against each other and against the possible risk that has to be accepted more complicated. Applied to the question of the DTC, Iserson summarizes the problem in the following way:

> [T]he question of whether physicians will report to and remain at work is really about the pivotal point when the *perception of risk* overwhelms professional values and duties. Morally speaking, when does the right to protect oneself from grave risks outweigh the duty to care for patients in need?
>
> (Iserson et al., 2008, p. 348, emphasis added)

Thus, as Clark proposes, on the one hand we have to lead "some discussion of what is meant by acceptable risk" (Clark, 2006, p. 170); and, on the other hand, during epidemics and other difficult situations it is necessary to aim for a realistic and objective risk assessment, in order not to rely on pure and biased perception. The latter is, however, difficult as during situations like epidemics "people will not be able to assess their true risks until accurate information replaces what they imagine the risks to be" (Iserson et al., 2008, p. 349).

Neglected/underdeveloped public health ethics focus

It has been much argued that public health and thus public health ethics should be the more important focus during epidemics. Benatar, for example, asserts that the EVD

> epidemic raises the necessity of extending the bioethics discourse beyond interpersonal ethics to the ethics of public health and the ethics of the international relations.
>
> (Benatar, 2015)

By spending too much energy for example questioning the authorization of experimental treatments or the use of new drugs, the risk is high that "Thousands died while we argued over the wrong questions" (Gericke, 2015). Instead, the focus should be that doctors care for a whole population and, in order to do so, leave the focus on individual clinical ethics. According to Dawson:

> If Ebola is to be controlled, it will be because of old-fashioned public health measures.... Ebola is a public health emergency, not an opportunity to just treat a few patients.
>
> (Dawson, 2015, p. 108)

Similarly, the debate around the DTC should also be led in a way to account for the collective aspects of the context during epidemics and thus at least be amended by the additional perspective of public health ethics.

Reciprocal duties vis-à-vis HCPs

A last point, which is worth being mentioned in the context of the duty to care, is the question of reciprocal duties of the society (or the patients) vis-à-vis doctors and HCPs. The basic formulation of the argument is that if we expect HCPs to accept the duty to work under a level of risk that is relatively higher during epidemics, then they can expect those who benefit to provide a commensurate recognition and fair compensation. Accordingly, the members of society (who all benefit from the HCPs' commitment) have a duty that is reciprocal to the duty to care of HCPs.[10] This societal duty could for example entail providing adequate means and resources to HCPs or adapting the remuneration to the higher risk.

Conclusion

In this chapter, we discussed the question whether doctors and HCP have a duty to care for patients when doing so exposes the caregivers to significant risks of harm—namely in the context of epidemics. The question was first restricted to an individual duty to care on the national level (which is the main concern in the literature) and then in the second section extended to the discussion of a state-centered and internationalized duty to care. The latter could be the moral justification for sending *military* health care personnel to treat epidemics abroad.

The review of the academic literature on the concept of a DTC proved that such a duty can be based on several arguments and be justified according to a variety of models. Thus, doctors indeed have a moral duty to care for patients and have to accept some risk of harm. Yet, objections against the DTC have to be taken into account and the duty is therefore neither unconditional nor without limits. More concretely, the basis and the scope of the DTC should be publicly discussed within society in order to evaluate public expectations about the professional duties of doctors and HCP (see Sokol, 2003) and to find a consent acceptable both for society and for the members of the medical professions. This is all the more important as such consent would serve to both strengthen the resulting duty to care as well as clearly spell out the limits of the DTC.

In the context of epidemics or *international* health emergencies, the addressee of the DTC can be extended to include states based on the principle of humanity or within the paradigm of the Responsibility to Protect. Rather selfish or at least egoistic arguments like the protection of their own citizens can be added. As a result, doctors and HCP who are employed by the state (and are thus state agents) inherit the state's duty to intervene in such situations. With regard to humanitarian missions during international epidemics, this argument is mainly relevant for the military medical services: states could thus legitimately rely on them in order to fulfill their duty to care abroad. As a result, humanitarian missions in regions affected by epidemics can be justified and military medical personnel, as state agents, be sent into such missions.

Acknowledgment

This research was supported by the Swiss Centre of Competence for Military and Disaster Medicine (Komp Zen MKM), which is funding the research conducted at the Zurich Center for Military Medical Ethics. The views expressed in this chapter are those of the author and do not necessarily represent or reflect the views of the funding body.

Notes

1 See also the definition and its discussion in the introduction to this volume.
2 We will not look into the historical development of such a duty in professional codes. This has been done, e.g., by Fox (1988), Sokol (2003), and Baker (2006).
3 See Malm, 2008. p. 164.
4 We will discuss the epistemic problem of defining risk briefly in a later section of this chapter.
5 With regard to military HCPs, it will be interesting to see whether they have a different obligation to take a higher risk because their "second profession" as soldier demands them to do so (see below).
6 The personal acceptance of such a DTC however depends on the individual character and the personality of the doctor or HCP. The latter statement does not imply an ethical argument, though.
7 www.icrc.org/eng/resources/documents/misc/fundamental-principles-commentary-010179.htm
8 Similar positions that highlight the special obligations of the wealthier countries vis-à-vis poorer people have been taken by Rid and Emanuel (2014a, 2014b).
9 www.euractiv.com/sections/fighting-diseases-challenges-ahead/german-government-readies-eu-white-helmet-force-combat (accessed January 28, 2016).
10 This questions has been discussed, for the Ebola context, e.g., by Yakubu, Folayan, Sani-Gwarzo, Nguku, Peterson, and Brown (2016).

References

Alexander, G. C. and Wynia, M. K. 2003. Ready and willing? Physicians' sense of preparedness for bioterrorism. *Health Affairs (Millwood)*, 22, 189–197.

Arras, J. D. 1988. The fragile web of responsibility: AIDS and the duty to treat. *The Hastings Center Report*, 18, 10–20.

Baker, R. 2006. Chapter 5: medical ethics and epidemics: a historical perspective. In J. Balint, S. Philpott, R. Baker and M. Strosberg (eds.) *Ethics and Epidemics* (pp. 93–133). Amsterdam: Elsevier.

Benatar, S. 2015. Explaining and responding to the Ebola epidemic. *Philosophy, Ethics, and Humanities in Medicine*, 10, 5.

Brody, H. and Avery, E. N. 2009. Medicine's duty to treat: pandemic illness solidarity and vulnerability. *Hastings Center Report*, 39, 40–48.

Clark, C. C. 2006. Chapter 7: doctors, duties, and dangers: the reasonable physician and contagious populations. In J. Balint, S. Philpott, R. Baker and M. Strosberg (eds.) *Ethics and Epidemics* (pp. 163–174). Amsterdam: Elsevier.

Daniels, N. 1991. Duty to treat or right to refuse? *Hastings Center Report*, 21, 36–46.

Dawson, A. J. 2015. Ebola: what it tells us about medical ethics. *Journal of Medical Ethics*, 41, 107–110.

Fox, D. M. 1988. The politics of physicians' responsibility in epidemics: a note on history. *The Hastings Center Report*, 18, 5–10.

Gericke, C. A. 2015. Ebola and ethics: autopsy of a failure. *BMJ*, 350, h2105.

Huber, S. J. and Wynia, M. K. 2004. When pestilence prevails physician responsibilities in epidemics. *American Journal of Bioethics*, 4, 5–11.

International Commission on Intervention and State Sovereignty, Evans, G. J., Sahnoun, M. and International Development Research Centre (Canada). 2001. *The Responsibility to Protect: Report of the International Commission on Intervention and State Sovereignty*. Ottawa: International Development Research Centre.

International Committee of the Red Cross (ICRC), World Medical Association (WMA), International Committee of Military Medicine (ICMM), International Council of Nurses (ICN) and International Pharmaceutical Federation (FIP). 2015. *Ethical Principles of Health Care in Times of Armed Conflict and Other Emergencies*. Geneva: ICRC.

Iserson, K. V., Heine, C. E., Larkin, G. L., Moskop, J. C., Baruch, J. and Aswegan, A. L. 2008. Fight or flight: the ethics of emergency physician disaster response. *Annals of Emergency Medicine*, 51, 345–353.

Malm, H., May, T., Francis, L. P., Omer, S. B., Salmon, D. A. and Hood, R. 2008. Ethics, pandemics, and the duty to treat. *American Journal of Bioethics*, 8, 4–19.

Médecins Sans Frontières. 2015. *Pushed to the Limit and Beyond. A Year into the Largest Ever Ebola Outbreak*. Geneva: Médecins Sans Frontières.

Rid, A. and Emanuel, E. J. 2014a. Ethical considerations of experimental interventions in the Ebola outbreak. *Lancet*, 384(9957), 1896–1899.

Rid, A. and Emanuel, E. J. 2014b. Why should high-income countries help combat ebola? *JAMA*, 312(13), 1297–1298.

Singer, P. 1972. Famine, affluence, and morality. *Philosophy and Public Affairs*, 1, 229–243.

Singer, P. A., Benatar, S. R., Bernstein, M., Daar, A. S., Dickens, B. M., MacRae, S. K., Upshur, R. E., Wright, L. and Shaul, R. Z. 2003. Ethics and SARS: lessons from Toronto. *BMJ*, 327, 1342–1344.

Sokol, D. K. 2003. *Healthcare Workers Duty to Care and Severe Infectious Diseases*. London: Imperial College Faculty of Medicine.

Sokol, D. K. 2006. Virulent epidemics and scope of healthcare workers' duty of care. *Emerging Infectious Diseases*, 12, 1238.

Wynia, M. K., Kurlander, J. F. and Green, S. K. 2006. Chapter 6: physician professionalism and preparing for epidemics: challenges and opportunities. In J. Balint, S. Philpott, R. Baker and M. Strosberg (eds.) *Ethics and Epidemics* (pp. 135–161). Amsterdam: Elsevier.

Yakubu, A., Folayan, M. O., Sani-Gwarzo, N., Nguku, P., Peterson, K. and Brown, B. 2016. The Ebola outbreak in Western Africa: ethical obligations for care. *Journal of Medical Ethics*, 42, 209–210.

Zuger, A. and Miles, S. H. 1987. Physicians, aids, and occupational risk: historic traditions and ethical obligations. *JAMA*, 258, 1924–1928.

10 Deploying military doctors to stem deadly epidemics

Paul Gilbert

Introduction

In September 2014 the president of Médecins Sans Frontières, Joanne Liu, said that it would require a major military mobilization to stop the spread of Ebola (Arie 2014, p. 16). It was, she said, not just equipment and logistical support that were needed but qualified and trained medical staff. Local doctors and volunteers were running out and only the military could be deployed in the numbers required at short notice. The environment which military doctors were being expected to enter in order to diagnose and treat Ebola patients was a very dangerous one. Many health workers had already died of a disease with a 50 per cent death rate. Yet Dr Liu took it for granted that states could reasonably order their military medical staff to provide medical assistance despite these risks. The question I am addressing in this chapter is what the justification for issuing such orders might be.

The reason why the president of MSF called for military assistance was that she wanted help from foreign states in the fight against Ebola in Africa. States can only act through their agents and the only agents of the state who can in practice be ordered to assist in this way are members of the armed forces. States can facilitate the deployment of civilian volunteers and this has been done quite widely in respect of Ebola in West Africa. In this case it is individuals who are providing help, albeit with the support of states, not the states themselves, which is only possible if appropriate members of their forces are deployed. In theory, states could have purely medical forces who are under orders in the same way as their military forces are, but whose task was to fight epidemics and so forth rather than wars. But in practice it is only military medical staff who can be ordered to do this, even though it is not their primary purpose. It is important to recognize that military doctors assisting in fighting epidemics are normally acting as agents of the state and not as individuals. This is evidently the case if they are under orders to so act, but it is also the case if they volunteer for such duties, since, unlike civilians, it is duties for which they volunteer and they remain within the military command structure in performing these duties. So, unless they are released from the command structure, they act as military men and women, and hence as agents of the state and not as individuals, in just the same way as other soldiers who volunteer for dangerous assignments. The risks they take are risks not only to themselves but to the force to which they belong, for their deaths would be a loss to that force of members with valuable skills and responsibilities. It is, however, only the risks to themselves that I shall be concerned with here, ignoring the question of whether a state can afford to expose its personnel to such risks.

Taking risks to tackle epidemics

How may we judge the level of risk that military medics should be required to take? To answer this question we first need to investigate what the role of a doctor within the military is. First, the role of a doctor is, so to speak, self-standing, like that of a philosopher, for example, in the sense that pursuing the calling is possible outside of any institution and is answerable to standards and requirements independent of the institution within which it may be pursued. Second, the role is pervasive in that a doctor is expected to give medical assistance in an emergency even outside of his or her employment. Third, it is autonomous in that the doctor is solely responsible for the medical judgements on which he or she acts and should not be ordered to act otherwise. This brings us to the relation between the military doctor's medical and military roles. The military employs doctors as doctors in the role just outlined, not as mere medical technicians to carry out the employers' demands irrespective of medical priorities, for this would offend against their autonomy, and it is, indeed, a consequence of their self-standing status.[1]

If this account is correct then we can see that we need a different answer to the question of what medical risk a military doctor should be prepared to face from that given to the question to what military risk they should be exposed. For it is surely a question of medical judgement alone what risk a doctor should confront in order to treat a patient, especially when it is a risk of a potentially fatal infection. The risk must enter the doctor's calculations in the same way that the risks to a patient of some medical intervention need to be assessed. Just as the latter requires the patient's informed consent, so in the former it is up to the doctor whether to determine whether to run a certain level of risk in order to provide treatment to an infected patient. We do indeed expect a certain degree of courage among doctors, but we do not expect self-sacrificial acts. It follows that military doctors as autonomous agents cannot properly be ordered to run medical risks in the line of duty that they consider unreasonable. There need to be, then, good reasons for exposing them to the risks involved in fighting epidemics.

To the question of what military risks military medics should be exposed to, we can return a different sort of answer, since it is a feature of the military calling that members of the armed forces are required to face whatever risks their orders expose them to. There are two levels at which the exposure to risk of military personnel, including military doctors, needs to be judged as reasonable or unreasonable. The obvious one is in the conduct of operations, where it is military commanders who must assess what risks are reasonable to take for the military objectives they aim to achieve in the campaign. The other level concerns whether the campaign should have been undertaken in the first place, and at this level it is the country's statesmen who must consider whether the employment of its forces is justified by their political goals, given the risks to which these forces will be exposed. The purposes for which the armed forces exist are principally military ones, but secondarily they may be expected to assist in civil emergencies such as floods and earthquakes, which threaten the lives and well-being of citizens as much as the hazards of war. By extension, then, we can regard the risks faced in such emergencies as military risks.

However, when we turn to assisting in emergencies like epidemics, military medics find themselves in a distinctly different position from that in which they are placed in war. In war their medical neutrality affords them protection from direct attack, though they may be the indirect victims of the enemy's military operations. But in an epidemic they are more, not less, exposed to danger than other troops. The danger is from one angle a medical risk, incurred in virtue of their medical role. But that they are deployed to a zone of danger is analogous to their being exposed to a military risk in virtue of their military calling. Yet, having been so deployed, it is, I contend, up to the medics to decide what risks to run in treating the epidemic's victims, and here a set of medical judgements will provide the reasons for their decisions. Thus politicians will have to take into account the military medics' attitude to these risks in deciding whether to deploy them, just as they take into account the views of senior soldiers about the risks of a war in deciding whether to embark upon it. In this connection we should note that greater risks may need to be taken in an epidemic than in treating a patient with a one-off illness. This is because of the public health dimension, whereby treating victims will help to halt the epidemic's spread and the greater the number of lives thereby saved will justify the greater risk. It is up to medics to make an agreed judgement here that will feed into the politicians' decisions on deployment.

Before looking at the kinds of justification a state might offer for sending its military medics abroad to assist in treating the victims of an epidemic, I want to contrast this case with other scenarios in which they might be exposed to the same sort of risk. The first is that in which the forces of which the medics are members are themselves affected by an epidemic. Here there can be no doubt that treating them is part of their expected duties so long as the risks do not outweigh the benefits. Similar considerations apply to a second sort of case in which doctors are clearly acting in a military capacity as well as a medical one. Here troops have occupied a territory and have responsibility for administering it and attending to the immediate needs of its people. If an epidemic breaks out it will be military medics who are looked to for treatment, and this case can be seen as an extension of their duty to treat sick POWs, for it is as a result of military action that the occupation has occurred and the people find themselves, in a sense, prisoners and dependants. A third case arises when an epidemic rages in one's own population and the civilian health services are unable to cope with it. This case resembles the civil emergencies mentioned earlier and, as there, it can be regarded as an extension of purely military duties. It can be so regarded in part because the state has an obligation to do what it can to secure the well-being of its citizens and will deploy what resources it has, including the military, to discharge this obligation. Those who sign up to the military understand this and, broadly speaking, accept the risks involved, which are generally less than more purely military ones. It is an apparently different matter, however, when we turn to consider the deployment of forces, including medics, to deal with epidemics abroad, and it is to the justification for this that we now turn.

Giving reasons for facing risks

The question of whether a state is justified in sending its military medics into a risky environment abroad to tackle an epidemic divides into two parts. First, we need to ask what reason a state may have for assisting another in treating its people. Second, we need to know whether it is justified in requiring its military doctors to take on the task, with all the risks to themselves that this entails. Both questions need to be addressed, for it is not enough simply to say that the state has a right to order any of its military personnel into any situation of potential danger, since this is what they have accepted in joining the forces. This is because the dangers they have accepted are principally military dangers and certain fairly obvious extensions of these. It is in their military role that they can legitimately be given orders and not as all-purpose servants of the state. Thus the reason why it is not enough to say that military medics should just do what they are ordered to do is that they should feel that they are being ordered to do something for an appropriate reason. That is to say, they should be able to think that in obeying these orders they are doing something they have a reason to do as performers of their role. Only if the state has the right sort of reasons for giving the orders will this be the case, so we need to ask what such reasons might be.

I am not saying that military doctors should be convinced by the state's justification any more than that a soldier needs to be convinced by the state's justification for every armed conflict into which they are thrust. I am saying that the state's justification for requiring its military agents to act in a certain way must be of an appropriate form to convince them in their role as soldiers etc. Thus, to justify a war on the grounds that it is waged to convert the enemy to one's religion does not have the appropriate form, since qua soldier, as this role is now understood, one's duties are secular and can be performed whatever one's religion. To appeal to religious reasons would be to appeal to the personal convictions of soldiers, not just to what they can be taken to accept simply as soldiers of the state they serve. They may be prepared to die for their religion, if they share the relevant conviction, but it is as believers that they die, not as soldiers. As soldiers they cannot properly be ordered to put their lives at risk for a faith they may not share. By contrast, a justification in terms of self-defence does have the appropriate form to give soldiers a reason to fight, since they can be taken to accept that the state they have signed up to serve is worth defending.

The general point is that when holders of a role are required to act in a certain way the reasons they are given must be ones they can appreciate as holders of the role. They cannot be reasons which would recommend themselves to the holders as individuals with their particular opinions and beliefs. Someone acting in a role must in principle be able to justify what they do in terms of the requirements and restrictions of the role, even if acting under orders within a hierarchical structure of authority as in the armed forces. Someone who acts on the basis of the wrong form of justification may not be acting as the relevant role-holder at all, as with the religious warrior. Similarly, a military medic who exposed him or herself to unreasonable risks to treat a patient would not be acting simply as a doctor but as a self-sacrificing individual, motivated by concerns above and beyond those that come with this role. It follows that a military medic could not legitimately be ordered to so act. We turn now, then, to what sort of consideration can properly figure in the reasons for ordering military medics abroad into the risky environment of an epidemic in order to treat its victims.

Tackling epidemics as humanitarian intervention

What I want to suggest is that the only acceptable justification for sending military doctors abroad to tackle epidemics takes the form of a plausible analogy between what they are conceived as doing there and what they would be doing in a clearly military operation. I shall start by looking at what I shall term the humanitarian intervention justification because it shares some features of the way in which sending troops into other counties to avert a humanitarian catastrophe is justified. Intervention does not need to be coercive and non-consensual: witness Nigeria's recent reliance on help from other states in its battle with Boko Haram to protect the Christian population of its country. This situation has parallels with that which occurred in Guinea, Liberia, and Sierra Leone, when those states found themselves unable to cope with an outbreak of Ebola without outside intervention. In both cases there was a humanitarian crisis and the military forces of other states were allowed into a country to ameliorate the situation and to prevent it from deteriorating further.

There are different ways of developing a humanitarian intervention justification, one of which we may term the cosmopolitan justification.[2] Such a justification asserts the existence of obligations of humanitarian assistance to people irrespective of their national identity, just as it is provided to compatriots. This sort of cosmopolitanism is gestured at in the report *Ethics and Ebola*, prepared by the American Presidential Commission for the Study of Bioethical Issues. The report asserts:

> Both health care professionals and members of the public feel the pull of moral obligations to respond with assistance in the face of profound human suffering. Such commitments are sometimes articulated in terms of what we owe to each other as members of a global community.[3]

However, this seems to be the wrong kind of reason to justify sending military medics abroad to fight epidemics. It is not what they feel as individuals about their moral obligations that is relevant here, but rather what their duty to do as military doctors can be. This is because, as indicated earlier, it is normally not as individuals but as military doctors deployed by their government that they find themselves having to cope with an epidemic. Appealing to individual moral beliefs provides the wrong sort of reason for them because they seemingly need not have these beliefs. Indeed, military doctors might as equally be nationalists as cosmopolitans, believing that as individuals they have moral obligations to their compatriots that outweigh any obligations to others. So the problem with cosmopolitanism is not that it is not true. It might be true and still not provide the right kind of justification – the kind that can in principle be accepted by military doctors simply in virtue of their holding this role.

Now this may be challenged by asserting that we now all do share a cosmopolitan mindset because we do live in a global community where obligations to others outside our state are readily accepted, as the Presidential Commission report maintains. The idea that we now live in a global community is intended to support cosmopolitanism in at least two ways. Psychologically, it suggests that we can think of ourselves citizens of the world rather than only of smaller units and can therefore accept wider obligations. Second, and morally, if the narrower obligations we have are taken to derive from the relationships we have to others then if we stand in relationships to others across the world that are in no way different ethically from more local ones then we have the same obligations to them too. However, it is very doubtful if there is in any literal sense such a community with its associated obligations. The reason is that it is a regime of rules which, however vague and unstated they may be, is what constitutes a community.[4] Without a regime of rules the supposed analogy between citizens of a state and so-called global citizens breaks down.[5] Citizenship of a state requires occupancy of a variety of roles, the correct performance of which is necessary for the community of the state to function properly. This is the point Aristotle makes by comparing citizenship to membership of a ship's crew, each of whom has a necessary function (Aristotle, III, iv). This comparison points up the difficulty in the idea of a global community; for, while we can see how proper performance of the ordinary roles in life contributes to the functioning of a city or a country, it is quite unclear what this would mean on a global scale. We may well have global obligations, but seeing these as springing from membership of a global community is arguably less than helpful.[6]

We may question the Presidential Commission report's sweeping claim that 'members of the public feel the pull of moral obligations' on a global scale. However, might it not be that 'health professionals' do feel this pull, at least with regard to the obligation to provide medical treatment, simply in virtue of their role? Are not doctors natural cosmopolitans, since they must be impartial in their treatment of the sick, giving priority to those in most medical need irrespective of their nationality? For military doctors this requirement is enshrined in the principle of medical neutrality as set out in the 1949 Geneva Convention and its 1977 Additional Protocols, namely that wounded soldiers and civilians should be treated without distinction as to their affiliation, but only in accordance with medical priorities.[7] This principle bears out the self-standing character of the doctor's role in the military: he or she is employed as a doctor with a doctor's priorities and the autonomy to act on them.[8] Does not this show that in their role as military doctors they evince cosmopolitan attitudes, such that a cosmopolitan justification of their deployment would be appropriate?

I do not think that this conclusion follows. The impartiality of military physicians shows only that if they are posted abroad they can have no reason not to treat the epidemic's victims if the risk is acceptable. It does nothing to show why they should be so posted. We must distinguish here between impartiality in the treatment of patients and impartiality in the selection of possible patients. Civilian doctors may well not be impartial in the selection of possible patients, perhaps by normally treating only private patients, even if others have greater medical needs. In the case of military doctors, their possible patients are selected for them. But that they must be impartial when treating such patients does nothing to show why they must be assigned such a risky group in the first place. A separate justification is needed for putting them in this position.

Another way of developing a humanitarian intervention justification for this is provided by the so-called society of states model of international relations.[9] Where there is a regime of rules, by contrast with its apparent absence in an alleged global community, is in relations between states. These do form a society, on this view, just because they expect from each other conformity to certain norms of behaviour. Some of these norms are codified in international law; others are not. What we need to ask is whether there is an expectation of assistance in the case an epidemic breaking out in a country which is unable to deal with it without the help of other states. Sufferers from an epidemic arguably have a right to medical care, as is implied by Article 25 of the UN Universal Declaration of Human Rights. In the first instance, they have a claim against their own state to have this right to treatment honoured. This state will be trying to honour its obligations in seeking assistance from other states if it cannot cope alone. But do other states have an obligation to help? Within the international society of states there does seem to be some expectation that states in a good position to do so will help, and in doing so they deliver the medical care to which sufferers have a right.

This line of thinking does, I believe, offer the best prospect of a justification for ordering military medics abroad to tackle an epidemic in terms of this being a form of humanitarian intervention. We can compare it with a forcible military intervention to prevent a genocide, which is regarded as allowable under international law and which may be expected of states capable of mounting it effectively. In both cases, the military personnel involved – ordinary soldiers in one case, military medics in the other – may view what they are doing as acting in a way that enables their state to fulfil its international responsibilities, and they can regard the risks they run as those that they have accepted as the sort of agents of the state that they are.

Tackling epidemics as self-defence

I turn now to a second type of justification for deploying military medics to areas abroad hit by epidemics. I call this the self-defence justification since it exploits the analogy between military self-defence and acting abroad to prevent an epidemic spreading to one's own land and affecting one's own people with effects as bad or worse than those of war. Since self-defence is a task in which military medics are typically involved, along with other troops, it may seem natural that they should be engaged in the parallel work of defending their own people from an epidemic, not just by treating them when they are affected, as we saw earlier, but by treating others in order to prevent their own people from becoming affected. Although, by contrast with the ordinary case of self-defence, medics are, so to speak, in the front line, with the normal relationship between the risks run by medics and other troops reversed, this does nothing to upset the analogy. Nor is there a conflict between their military and their medical roles, since, just as military doctors can think of themselves in the normal case as both relieving suffering and getting troops back into action against an enemy, so in an epidemic they can credit themselves both with the relief of suffering and with stopping contagion spreading to their own people. Thus, on the self-defence justification, military doctors can regard their deployment abroad in an epidemic as expressing the way in which as military personnel they are defending their compatriots, but from a threat of a different kind from that in the normal case.

What sort of justification is this? The report *Ethics and Ebola* mentioned earlier states: 'Infectious disease epidemics ... are a matter of US and global concern for both ethical and prudential reasons'. After offering the humanitarian justification we have looked at, the report asserts that

> the second rationale for US engagement in global health emergencies, including the current epidemic, is prudentially based, that is, serving individual and collective interests. Given the capacity of infectious diseases to travel easily in an interconnected world and to destabilize regions and countries, epidemics must be addressed at their source.

The report goes on: 'Responding to outbreaks at their epicenter can be conceptualized in terms of enlightened self-interest ... given that individual or national interests are tied to the interests of others'.[10]

However, this dichotomy between the ethical and the prudential seems to me to be both misguided and dangerous. It is misguided because it presupposes too narrow a view of the responsibility of the state to its citizens, namely as simply that of pursuing their individual interests more or less effectively. But we do surely think of the relation between state and citizen in more ethical terms, regarding a state that fails to look after its citizens properly as failing morally, that is to say, that its leaders are failing morally. They are failing morally because they are not fulfilling the obligations that flow from the trust that citizens place in them as leaders of the state. To fail to protect them from infection where this is possible would be an example of this. I want to say, then, that we can properly regard posting military medics abroad to protect the population at home as having an ethical justification in virtue of this aim alone, and not a merely prudential one.

I have tried to show that the idea that the self-defence justification is only prudential is misguided. I also said that it is dangerous. It is dangerous because it suggests that these reasons might easily be trumped by genuinely ethical considerations. This may literally demoralize military medics, for example those who are kept at home in their own state in case infection spreads there when there is a greater medical need elsewhere. But these medics should be able to see what they are doing as having an ethical justification, albeit a different one, just as a more purely humanitarian deployment has an ethical justification. In speaking of military medics as being able to think of what they are doing as ethically justified I do not mean that it chimes with their individual ethical beliefs. This, as I have claimed earlier, would be irrelevant to the sort of reasons for which they should act as military medics. Rather, I mean that they should be able to think that simply through the correct performance of this dual role they are acting ethically.

It is not for military medics in general to decide where they should be sent and thus who their possible patients should be. That is a decision to be taken high up in the military and political command chain, albeit with the advice of senior medical officers. However, military doctors on the ground need to feel that they are acting for good reasons in terms of their professional medical ethics, and the idea that some course of action they may be ordered to take is merely prudential stands in the way of their sense of acting ethically.

Yet there may still seem to be a conflict here between the military and the medical aspects of a military doctor's role if he or she is not sent where there is the greatest medical need because being elsewhere better serves to protect their own people. I do not think that there is, for the disposition of these doctors is still serving the purposes of public health. Doctors in general usually care for their own patients, only occasionally having to treat emergencies that arise elsewhere. It is only in such cases that they may be expected to desert their own patients to go where medical need is greater. The patients of military doctors are those assigned to them by the military command, be they their own compatriots or victims abroad. Wherever they are, military doctors should be able to use their medical judgement to determine their immediate priorities. So long as this is the case they need not feel that as doctors they are not fulfilling their obligations if they are ordered elsewhere than where there is greatest medical need. As individuals they may not agree with that decision, but the form that the justification of it takes in terms of self-defence can satisfy them that as military doctors they are properly performing their role.

In conclusion, then, I think that both the humanitarian intervention and the self-defence justifications for ordering military doctors abroad to treat the victims of epidemics can, if correctly formulated, give them good reasons for doing this work despite the risks. In many cases, both types of justification will apply, and military doctors will be able to think of themselves as both addressing important medical priorities and protecting their own compatriots from a deadly threat.

Notes

1 For development of these points see Gilbert (2013).
2 I discuss cosmopolitan justifications in Gilbert (2002).
3 Gutmann, 2015, p. 4. Among those who see the issue in these terms is Dawson (2015).
4 It is not enough to say that 'what is distinctive of community is some feeling of solidarity' so that 'a world community exists when people acknowledge a global obligation to help each other when times are hard' (Van Hooft 2009, pp. 142–143). For it is not just feelings but actual relationships of interdependence that constitute a community.
5 For a defence see Dower (2003).
6 For further development see Gilbert (2008).
7 See Gilbert (2014).
8 This does not conflict with their duties as members of the military, as I argue in Gilbert (2013, pp. 87–89).
9 This idea was pioneered by Bull (1977).
10 Gutmann (2015, pp. 4–6).

References

Arie, S. 2014. Without more troops we will not get the Ebola epidemic under control. *British Medical Journal*, 349, 16–18.

Aristotle. *Politics* (many editions).

Bull, H. 1977. *The Anarchical Society*. London: Macmillan.

Dawson, A. 2015. Ebola: what it tells us about medical ethics. *Journal of Medical Ethics*, 41(1), 107–110.

Dower, N. 2003. *An Introduction to Global Citizenship*. Edinburgh: Edinburgh University Press.

Gilbert, P. 2002. Repression, Secession and Intervention. In M. Moseley and R. Norman (eds) *Human Rights and Military Intervention*. Aldershot: Ashgate.

Gilbert, P. 2008. Global civil society and international morality. *The Philosophical Yearbook*, 21, 324–332.

Gilbert, P. 2013. Medical Neutrality and the Dilemmas of War. In M. L. Gross and D. Carrick (eds) *Military Medical Ethics for the 21st Century* (pp. 84–95). Farnham: Ashgate.

Gilbert, P. 2014. Medical neutrality. In D. Messelken and D. Winkler (eds) *Proceedings of the 4th ICMM Workshop on Military Medical Ethics* (pp. 10–23). Bern: Bundespublikationen.

Gutmann, A., Wagner, J. W., Allen, A. L., Arras, J. D., Atkinson, B. F., Farahany, N. A., Grady, C., Hauser, S. L., Kucherlapati, R. S., Michael, N. L. and Sulmasy, D. P. 2015. *Ethics and Ebola: Public Health Planning and Response*. Washington, DC: US Government.

Van Hooft, S. 2009. *Cosmopolitanism*. Stocksfield: Acumen.

Index

Page numbers in **bold** indicate figures.

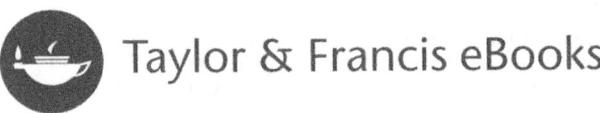
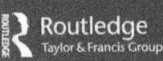